Contemporary Pediatric and Adolescent Sports Medicine

Series Editor
Lyle J. Micheli

Alexis C. Colvin • James N. Gladstone
Editors

The Young Tennis Player

Injury Prevention and Treatment

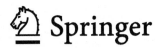 Springer

Editors
Alexis C. Colvin, MD
Department of Orthopaedic Surgery
Mount Sinai Medical Center
New York, NY
USA

James N. Gladstone, MD
Department of Orthopaedic Surgery
Mount Sinai Medical Center
New York, NY
USA

ISSN 2198-266X   ISSN 2198-2678   (electronic)
Contemporary Pediatric and Adolescent Sports Medicine
ISBN 978-3-319-27557-4   ISBN 978-3-319-27559-8   (eBook)
DOI 10.1007/978-3-319-27559-8

Library of Congress Control Number: 2016932528

Printed on acid-free paper

This Springer imprint is published by Springer Nature
The registered company is Springer International Publishing AG Switzerland

The Micheli Center for Sports Injury Prevention

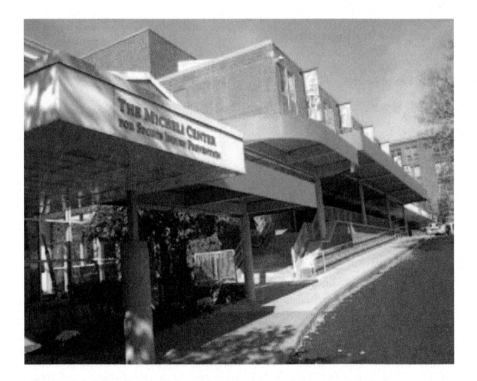

The mission of the Micheli Center for Sports Injury Prevention is at the heart of the Contemporary Pediatric and Adolescent Sports Medicine series.

The Micheli Center uses the most up-to-date medical and scientific information to develop practical strategies that help young athletes reduce their risk of injury as they prepare for a healthier future. The clinicians, scientists, activists, and technologists at the Micheli Center advance the field of sports medicine by revealing current injury patterns and risk factors while developing new methods, techniques, and technologies for preventing injuries.

The Micheli Center had its official opening in April 2013 and is named after Lyle J. Micheli, one of the world's pioneers in pediatric and adolescent sports medicine. Dr. Micheli is the series editor of Contemporary Pediatric and Adolescent Sports Medicine.

Consistent with Dr. Micheli's professional focus over the past 40 years, the Micheli Center conducts world-class medical and scientific research focused on the prevention of sports injuries and the effects of exercise on health and wellness. In addition, the Micheli Center develops innovative methods of promoting exercise in children.

The Micheli Center opens its doors to anyone seeking a healthier lifestyle, including those with medical conditions or illnesses that may have previously limited their abilities. Fellow clinicians, researchers, and educators are invited to collaborate and discover new ways to prevent, assess, and treat sports injuries.

Series Editor Biography

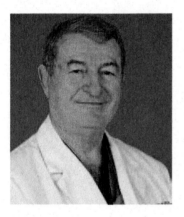

Dr. Lyle J. Micheli is the series editor of Contemporary Pediatric and Adolescent Sports Medicine. Dr. Micheli is regarded as one of the pioneers of pediatric and adolescent sports medicine, a field he has been working in since the early 1970s when he co-founded the USA's first sports medicine clinic for young athletes at Boston Children's Hospital.

Dr. Micheli is now Director of the Division of Sports Medicine at Boston Children's Hospital and Clinical Professor of Orthopedic Surgery at Harvard Medical School. He is a Past President of the American College of Sports Medicine and is currently the Secretary General for the International Federation of Sports Medicine. Dr. Micheli co-chaired the International Olympic Committee consensus on the health and fitness of young people through physical activity and sport.

In addition to many other honors, Dr. Micheli has served as Chairperson of the Massachusetts Governor's Committee on Physical Fitness and Sports, on the Board of Directors of the United States Rugby Football Foundation, as Chairman of the USA Rugby Medical and Risk Management Committee, and on the advisory board of the Bay State Games. He has been the Attending Physician for the Boston Ballet since 1977 and is Medical Consultant to the Boston Ballet School.

Dr. Micheli received his undergraduate degree from Harvard College in 1962 and his medical degree from Harvard Medical School in 1966. As an undergraduate student, Dr. Micheli was an avid athlete, competing in rugby, gridiron football, and boxing. Since graduating, Dr. Micheli has played prop for various Rugby clubs including the Boston Rugby Football Club, the Cleveland Blues Rugby Football Club, Washington Rugby Club, and Mystic Valley Rugby Club where he also served as team coach.

Dr. Micheli has authored over 300 scientific articles and reviews related to sports injuries, particularly in children. His present research activities focus on the prevention of sports injuries in children. Dr. Micheli has edited and authored several major books and textbooks.

Series Editor Foreword

I am a passionate advocate of sports for our young citizens. It is the main reason I pursued a career in sports medicine. Thanks to the health benefits and pure enjoyment they provide us, I am especially supportive of sports that can be played throughout our lives.

Of all the sports we can play in our childhood and youth, almost none has the same potential for lifetime participation as tennis.

It is for that reason that we need to help prevent injuries in our young tennis players and, if and when an injury does occur, to help those players get back on court as soon as possible. The player who has a happy and healthy tennis experience as a youngster is more likely to play as an adult – and even into senior citizenhood!

Therefore it gives me great pleasure to introduce this fine book by Drs. Colvin and Gladstone.

A review of the table of contents shows us that this is a comprehensive review of the subject matter, and reading the chapters themselves makes one understand that in these pages there is depth as well as breadth. I am especially impressed by the attention they have given to "overuse" injuries, which have become particularly problematic in sports where there is a lot of repetitive training. This book is a very important contribution to the literature.

Great young tennis players display artistry and athleticism, and we are privileged to watch them display their craft. I have no doubt that many of those players will get the benefit of the information in these pages. Just as important is to celebrate and care for the nonelite young tennis players who may not rise to exalted competitive heights but whose love of the game will stay with them. So that they are more likely to be sports-active throughout their lives, we need to keep all of our young athletes healthy!

Lyle J. Micheli, MD
Series Editor – Contemporary Pediatric and Adolescent Sports Medicine
O'Donnell Family Professor of Orthopaedic Sports Medicine
Boston Children's Hospital, Boston, MA, USA
Director, Division of Sports Medicine
Boston Children's Hospital, Boston, MA, USA
Clinical Professor of Orthopaedic Surgery
Harvard Medical School, Boston, MA, USA

Foreword

Can sport save society?

We certainly hope so. The United States of America is in the midst of an unprecedented health crisis. The facts are alarming. We are the second fattest country on the planet. For the first time in history, this generation of 10 and under kids is expected to die 5 years younger than their parents. National, regional, and local advertising campaigns have shifted our behavior in unhealthy ways. Our medical system does not promote preventative care: only 5 % of health-care expenditures are devoted to this critically important part of health-care delivery in this country.

To make matters worse, the United States has become one of the most physically illiterate countries in the developed world. Physical literacy is the ability, confidence, and desire to be physically active for life, and physical literacy provides a foundation for wellness through exercise. Why does this matter? There is strong evidence that exercise improves cardiorespiratory endurance, muscular fitness, favorable body composition, improved bone health, and improved cardiovascular and metabolic health biomarkers. Regular exercise reduces symptoms of anxiety and depression. Exercise facilitates synaptic plasticity in the hippocampus and improves cognition. Yet despite this concrete evidence, three out of every four high school students do not engage in the recommended amount of physical activity, and nearly 50 % of children are not provided a proper environment – in school or in public spaces – to develop the necessary foundation for lifelong exercise. These alarming statistics point to a country that is in crisis, a crisis that even threatens our national security.

Sport can be the answer or can further amplify what is wrong with our society. There is an exciting synergy in the sport world that may help assure that sport does indeed become an answer for our society. For example, the 48 National Governing Bodies of the United States Olympic Committee (USOC) and the National Collegiate Athletic Association (NCAA) have embraced the USOC's American Development Model, which provides a strategic pathway for sport from youth to high school to college and beyond. This model advocates for youth sport to occur in a fun and engaging atmosphere, with a focus on motor and foundational skill development, activities that are within the mental and physical reach of the child, multisport participation, and opportunities for either lifelong sport participation or for future elite athletes to maximize their potential. The Aspen Institute's Project Play identifies eight promising strategies that everyone can use to help every child become physically active in sport. Project Play's goal is for every child in America to be physically literate by age 12 through a fun and engaging pathway in sport whose core principles are as follows: (1) Ask kids what they want; (2) reintroduce free play; (3) encourage sport sampling; (4) revitalize in-town leagues; (5) think small; (6) design for development; (7) train all coaches; and (8) emphasize prevention.

The United States Tennis Association (USTA) is uniquely poised to provide a healthy pathway of sport for life and an elite pathway for college and professional tennis players through their comprehensive and holistic approach that embraces a phenomenal grassroots program with a comprehensive coaching education initiative. Tennis is a model sport for life, one that teaches individual skills and team competition and equally supports male and female development. The USTA not only understands the American Development Model and the core principles of Project Play but also provides the necessary foundation to make both a reality. Tennis has stepped up to address our societal woes.

As the Chief Medical Officer of the USTA, Alexis Colvin is uniquely positioned to guide us in how to assure that we get tennis right. And she has partnered with James Gladstone, who provides key sports medicine services to American tennis players. Yes, tennis is part of the solution for our society, but like any sport, tennis must foster an environment of injury prevention and proper treatment. *The Young Tennis Player: Injury Prevention and Treatment* has arrived at just the right moment. This essential book is filled with the wisdom and insight to help assure that America's tennis players are provided the opportunity to excel for life. Yes, sport can save society, and tennis is a key ingredient. Drs. Colvin and Gladstone provide an important recipe for getting it right.

Brian Hainline, MD
NCAA Chief Medical Officer
Clinical Professor of Neurology
New York University School of Medicine, New York, NY, USA
Indiana University School of Medicine, Indianapolis, IN, USA

Contents

Contributors

Steven M. Andelman, MD Department of Orthopaedic Surgery, Mount Sinai Medical Center, New York, NY, USA

Deena C. Casiero, MD Primary Care Sports Medicine, ProHEALTH Care Associates, Lake Success, NY, USA

Alexis C. Colvin, MD Department of Orthopaedic Surgery, Mount Sinai Medical Center, New York, NY, USA

James N. Gladstone, MD Department of Orthopaedic Surgery, Mount Sinai Medical Center, New York, NY, USA

Daniel Gould, PhD Kinesiology, Institute for the Study of Youth Sports, Michigan State University, East Lansing, MI, USA

Michael Hausman, MD Department of Orthopaedic Surgery, Mount Sinai Medical Center, New York, NY, USA

Andrew C. Hecht, MD Department of Spine Surgery, Mount Sinai Health System, New York, USA

Mount Sinai Spine Center, New York, USA

Steven M. Koehler, MD Department of Orthopaedic Surgery, Mount Sinai Medical Center, New York, NY, USA

Mark S. Kovacs, PhD, FACSM, CSCS*D, CTPS, MTPS Life Sport Science Institute and Department of Sport Health Science, Life University, Marietta, GA, USA

Steven Mcanany, MD Department of Orthopaedic Surgery, Mount Sinai Medical Center, New York, USA

Kristen M. Meier, MD Department of Orthopaedic Surgery, Mount Sinai Medical Center, New York, NY, USA

Jennifer Nalepa Kinesiology, Institute for the Study of Youth Sports, Michigan State University, East Lansing, MI, USA

Satoshi Ochi, MA, CSCS, RSCC*D, CTPS, MTPS USTA Player Development Incorporated, Boca Raton, FL, USA

Anne Pankhurst, PhD, BSc Organisation Name, Castle Cary, Somerset, UK

Diana Patterson, MD Resident Orthopaedic Surgery, Mount Sinai Medical Center, New York, USA

Ellen S. Rome, MD, MPH Center for Adolescent Medicine, Cleveland Clinic, Cleveland, OH, USA

Department of General Pediatrics, Cleveland Clinic Children's Hospital, Cleveland, OH, USA

Sarah E. Strandjord, BS Cleveland Clinic Lerner College of Medicine of Case Western University, Cleveland, OH, USA

Steve Wang, MD Kaiser Permanente Moanalua Medical Center, Hawaii, USA

Steven B. Weinfeld, MD Foot and Ankle Service, Mount Sinai Medical Center, New York, NY, USA

Chapter 1
10u Tennis: The Essentials of Developing Players for the Future

Anne Pankhurst

Introduction

Many sport organizations have realized that their sport needs to be adapted and adjusted for young children, simply because children have different physical, mental, emotional, social and competitive needs and abilities. In this respect, tennis has been no different. In the 1970s, Sweden developed a format of the game that was found to be very suitable for young children under 10. It was called Short Tennis, probably because it used a smaller court, a short plastic racquet and a foam ball. The format was adopted in the UK very quickly. It developed to become Mini Tennis in which the equipment changed in size as the children got older and increased in height. It included larger courts, shorter and lighter racquets (in comparison to adult racquets) and a range of felt balls that increased in speed and bounce height to correspond to the increasing height and strength of 10u children as they grew taller and stronger.

From the mid-1990s, Mini Tennis became the way in which children aged 10 and under learned to play tennis across much of Europe. The International Tennis Federation (ITF) promoted Mini Tennis as Tennis 10's across the world, and an increasing number of nations began to use both the format and the equipment to start all 10u players in the game. A number of research projects [1–3] endorse the use of different court sizes and low compression balls as contributing positively to the success rate of 10u children in terms of developing tennis strokes and movement.

However, what had become common practise in many countries was not part of tennis in the USA until 2006. Further, initial resistance to the 10u equipment and smaller courts in specific areas of the nation was evident. Such resistance was

A. Pankhurst, PhD, BSc
4 Yeablseys Way, Ansford, Castle Cary BA7 7HB, Somerset, UK
e-mail: anne@annepankhurst.co.uk

© Springer International Publishing Switzerland 2016
A.C. Colvin, J.N. Gladstone (eds.), *The Young Tennis Player: Injury Prevention and Treatment,* Contemporary Pediatric and Adolescent Sports Medicine,
DOI 10.1007/978-3-319-27559-8_1

1

perhaps understandable in a nation that had produced many tennis champions over the years, using full size courts and adult equipment irrespective of the age of the player. However, in 2012, the ITF changed the rules of the sport to make slower balls and smaller courts required practise for 12 and under tennis. The outcome of the rule change in the USA was a real push by the United States Tennis Association (USTA) for tennis coaches, teachers and parents to adopt good practise and teach tennis to 10u children using the modified equipment and courts. As of yet, despite the ITF rule change and the work of USTA, the acceptance of change still meets some pockets of resistance, but it is fair to say that the tide has turned and the 10u tennis format and equipment is used extensively to develop young tennis players across the USA. USTA, in a similar manner to other nations, has two key objectives for 10u tennis: to increase participation in the sport and to develop the potential of every child.

This chapter will first outline what 10u tennis is and identify how it differs from adult tennis. It will then discuss how and why the developmental processes that young children go through affects their ability to learn and compete in the sport. It will consider the role of parents, coaches and the organizational structure in the changes that 10u tennis brings. The purpose of the chapter is to highlight the emerging need for synergy between the developmental process of every child and the behaviour of parents, coaches and the organizers of the sport if USTA's twin objectives are to be realized. The thesis is that an absence of synergy does exist and if it persists will reduce both the opportunities for long-term participation in the sport and the chances of developing future world class players.

An Overview of 10 and Under Tennis

It was noted earlier that many sports have realized the difficulties and even impossibilities of young children participating fully in many adult sport environments. The road to success for young children is unlikely if they play on adult fields, courts or arenas with equipment that is too large, too heavy or too fast for them to handle while trying to compete in adult-style competition. Common sense has prevailed: different sports have made adaptations for children. As examples, baseball has T ball, football has flag football and junior soccer uses a smaller and lighter ball and (sometimes) a smaller field. All have junior competitive structures where children play for shorter time periods and often in smaller teams.

In a similar way, tennis has adapted the court areas, balls and racquets to make them more appropriate for 10u children. The adaptations are progressive, 'colour-coded' and relate to the chronological age of the child. Thus, 5–8-year-olds play with foam or red felt balls on a 36×18 feet court with a lower net. They use a light, short racquet between 17 and 23 inches in length. 8–9-year-olds, being taller, play with a (faster) orange felt ball, on a 60×21 feet court with a racquet that is between 23 and 25 inches in length. 9–10-year-olds play with a (even faster) green felt ball on a full size (78×27 feet) court, using a racquet that is between 25 and 26 inches.

Finally, by the age of 11 or 12, most young players are able to play with the fast yellow (adult) ball on a full-size court and use a full-size racquet.

From the details above, a principal issue can be identified: as children get older they are able to cope with different equipment, faster balls and larger court areas. This is because they grow in size and strength and are able to move faster. We also know that young children are smaller, have slower reactions and less strength and speed than older children, so in the context of scale, the progressive adaptations outlined make sense. As an example, we know that young children improve both their reaction speed and their ability to 'track' an incoming ball as they get older and gain experience: thus, they can increasingly cope with a faster ball that bounces higher. The use of the different balls in 10u tennis is probably the most important change from the adult game. The compression of each colour ball is different: each travels at a different speed through the air and has a different bounce height thus helping young players gain skills and experience as they get older.

The link between colour-coded 10u equipment and the different court sizes is also important: the slower red ball is used on the red (smallest) court, the faster orange on the orange court and the fastest green ball on the green court. The court size itself is linked to the average leg and stride length and height of the child. Therefore, any increase in court size should be proportional and relate to the development of the child. In tennis, it is important that the player can cover the width and length of the court to get to the ball in the time frame that is available. However, while a 6' tall adult can typically move from the centre line to the side line on a full-size court in 3.5 strides, a 4'6" child will need 4.7 strides to do so. By playing on an orange court that same child will be able to get to the sideline in 3.5 strides.

In tennis, the length of the court is also important, because it decides the server's position in relation to the net. A small child on the full court baseline is too far from the net and too short in relation to it to serve the ball effectively. The child inevitably adapts the technique and so learns to hit the ball in an upwards 'loop' action just to get it over the net. Adults, in contrast, because of their height, can hit the serve on a downwards trajectory into the service court.

This overview has highlighted the adaptations to equipment and court areas that tennis has made for 10u children. However, in tennis, as in other sports, there are other elements of the adult game that need to be changed if they are to meet the needs of young children. As an example, tennis matches have no fixed timelines. Thus, 10u tennis uses abbreviated scoring procedures so that matches are shorter and competitive time frames are more suitable for 10u children. As an example, on a red court, the players may play one game to seven points (or the best of three games to seven points), and on an orange court may play the first to four games in a three-set match. 10u matches can also run for a specific time with the player who is ahead when the allocated time is up being the winner.

The changes outlined above indicate the willingness of USTA as the tennis organization in the USA to adapt elements of the sport to meet the *needs* of young children as a group. However, a number of other factors also affect the *ability* of these same children to learn and compete in the sport. The next section examines in more detail why the abilities of different children should also be a major reason in deciding which equipment and system individual children should use. It thus begins to examine the issue of synergy.

It is apparent that, despite the best efforts of USTA, a lack of synergy does appear to exist – and is increasing – between the abilities of young children as individuals and the practises which coaches, parents and the USTA (as the organizer of the sport) currently employ. Thus, a closer examination of these practises – which link to the development of 10u children – could inform the discussion on the need for synergy between the realities of 10u children and current practise of coaches, parents and tennis organizers.

How and Why the Development of Young Players Affects Their Ability to Learn and Compete in Tennis

Growth, Maturation and Development of 10u Players

The previous section noted that the fundamental reasons for the adaptations to courts and equipment is that 10u children are continually growing, maturing and developing: 5-year-olds are not of the same size and height as 10-year-olds nor do they have the same level of maturity. As a result – and for positive reasons – the adaptations are progressive and they correspond to the chronological age of the child. Nonetheless, it is also obvious that the adaptations are 'across the board' for all children at a specific age and do not take individuality into account. They are thus based on the assumption that the processes of growth, maturation and development are identical in nature, timing and outcome for all children of the same chronological age. By implication, the needs and abilities of every child of the same age are considered to be identical. The information that follows will suggest that the processes of growth, maturation and development are, in fact, individual to every child, and for real progress to be made, they need to be considered.

Research [4, 5] suggests, and common sense verifies, that every person progresses through a number of recognized developmental stages from birth to old age: childhood, prepuberty, puberty, post-puberty and adulthood, as they grow and mature. In the specific context of 10u tennis, players are aged between five and ten, so for the majority of them, childhood is their predominant stage of development. We know [4] that during childhood, children typically grow steadily and at a rate of 2–3 inches per year. We also know that tennis organizations and coaches have agreed which courts and equipment are applicable to different ages of children based on each age groups' average size and height. Of great importance is the fact that competitive structures are also based around these same courts and equipment. Thus, all 5–8-year-olds compete on 'red' courts with red balls, all 8–9-year-olds on 'orange' courts and orange balls and all 9–10-year-olds on 'green' courts with green balls, each time with the appropriate length racquet.

However, this organizational 'neatness' ignores the fact that children are very individual in the timing of their growth and subsequent increase in height [6]. It is possible, therefore, that a child may be playing on the 'wrong' court for his or her actual height and size simply because he or she – as an individual – is either taller (or shorter) than the average for the age group. Reference to the normal curve of distribution of growth for children indicates a wide variety of heights for the same chronological age group! Further, there are two occasions when a more rapid increase in growth can occur before 10 years of age and thus add additional reasons why court size by chronological age can be problematic. The first is in the 'mini' growth spurt that some children go through around 8–9 years of age, clearly making an individual child taller than others of the same age. The second has a potentially much greater impact on the practise of allocating specific-sized courts and equipment to particular age groups, especially in a multicultural nation such as the USA. In essence, while the *pattern* of growth is known to be the same in that each child moves through the same stages as every other child, the *tempo* (rate) and *timing* of that growth is specific to the individual child. Research [7] indicates firstly a reduction in the age (timing) of the onset of puberty for both boys and girls in recent years and secondly notes a difference in the age at which puberty begins for different ethnic groups. Some children are known to experience their pubertal growth spurt around the age of 9 or 10 or even younger: i.e. within the 10u timeframe. Further, children in different ethnic groups are now known to begin the pubertal growth spurt at an earlier age than other groups. Finally, while the earlier age of maturation between boys and girls has been understood for many years, in 10u tennis, both genders play on the same-size court.

Clearly, all these factors impact the relationship between age and court/equipment size in 10u tennis. They thus potentially contribute to the issue of synergy between the children themselves and the system that has developed the current rules for courts and equipment for 10u children.

It is important to distinguish between the processes of growth, development and maturation in children and to understand their impact. Growth is defined as the natural process whereby a child increases in stature (height), weight and body size from birth to adulthood. Growth is clearly observable. As a result, it is perhaps easy to understand the 'allegiance' of sport organizations to what can be seen and measured when deciding equipment and court sizes for children of different ages.

Maturation is defined as the timing and progression of the skeletal, physiological, sexual and (importantly) emotional systems of young people as they progress through the different stages from childhood to adulthood [8]. Problematically, much of maturation is inferred rather than measurable. For example, physiological changes lead to increases in speed and strength and hormonal changes bring changes in sexual maturation while emotional development contributes to behavioural change [9]. Clearly, maturation contributes to change in young children, but it may not link linearly to growth and the increase in height. Certainly the different aspects of maturation contribute to the principles underpinning the 10u framework, but how they are implemented is important.

Development is the overarching factor that links all of the child's cognitive, emotional and social progress with growth and neuromuscular and sexual maturation. However, research and experience indicates that development again is not necessarily linearly linked with growth and maturation. A child can, for example, be taller than his or her peers, but lack the cognitive, emotional or social maturity to compete. Thus, even from the definitions given earlier, it is clear that there are practical issues in linking chronological age to court sizes and competitive structures. In simple terms:

1. Growth, maturation and development impact everything concerned with the training of children and young people in sports – and thus tennis.
2. Different abilities and skills do not develop in a linear manner. For example, while a 6-year-old may be taller and stronger than another 6-year-old, cognitively and emotionally, the same child could be 4 or even 8 years of age.

From the system and organizational perspective, it is the *expected* height and size of a particular age group that decides the court size, racquet and ball that will be used by those children. In the same way, it could be supposed that the *expected* level of emotional and cognitive development at different ages would decide competitive structures for a particular age group. As it will become clear, this is not the case. By the same token, the amount, type and timing of coaching, practise, training and competition on each court size should also link to chronological age. Again, there are concerns.

The reality is that not all children are the same. If all 10u players of the same chronological age do not develop, grow, mature and develop at the same rate and time, the inevitable question arises about the negative outcomes of current practise for individual players and ultimately for the organizational objectives.

The differences noted so far in this section have linked to the growth, maturation and development of 10u players. Other issues arise in terms of systems for 10u children in tennis: they are considered in turn in the next sections.

The Different Ages of 10u Players

Research indicates a number of important and different 'ages' for young children. They are not so important when working with older children or at all with adults. Reference has already been made to chronological age: the age on the child's birth certificate. This is clearly an easily identifiable age and one that is used consistently and constantly in junior sports, especially in competition. At this juncture, it is perhaps worth noting that adult sport rarely uses chronological age for competition!

In 10u tennis, the use of red, orange and green balls and court sizes is clearly tied (in organizational terms), to the *chronological age* of young players. So, 5–8-year-old players practise and play on the red court with red balls and the shortest racquets simply because they are aged 5–8.

However, the discussion on growth, maturation and development made it clear that some children are of a different *biological age* (*growth and maturity*) [9] than their peers. As a result, it may be inappropriate for a particularly tall 9-year-old to play on an orange court because in terms of height, he or she is a 10-year-old and is too tall for the orange court. Crucially, however cognitively, emotionally or even socially, that same 9-year-old may be of a different *developmental age* and so find it difficult (and unenjoyable) to play with 10-year-olds whom he or she does not know.

Relative age is another important 'age' to consider when working with young children. This refers to the month of the year (academic or sport) in which the child was born. *Relative age* [10] again impacts the abilities of individual children in different ways. This is because a child born at the beginning of a particular year is developmentally many months older than a child born at the end of that same year. So although the children are of the same *chronological age*, relatively, one is almost a year older than the other. *Relative age* will logically be of greater importance the younger the children are. 10u tennis is about young children, and so *relative age* is more important than it is for 17-year-olds. It will have an impact on the ability of every child, whether positively or negatively, and so again could conflict with policies that place children in chronological age groups.

In terms of the different 'ages' of children, while tennis organizations adopt sound principles regarding court sizes and equipment for a specific *chronological age* groups, other 'ages' may make the application of this principle somewhat questionable. Age is therefore another conundrum that will be discussed in the issue of synergy later in the chapter.

The Physical/Athletic Development of 10u Children

The discussion on growth, development and maturation in relation to 10u players highlighted the reality of differences between children of the same chronological age. Clearly, in their time in 10u tennis, not only are children growing, maturing and developing, but are also becoming more coordinated, stronger and faster. They are, in short, more able to perform different physical and athletic – and therefore sport – skills more easily. In any sport, physical and athletic ability is a major contributor to progress and success. In the tennis context, these skills underpin the technical skills to play the game and move around the court.

The acronym ABC'ss is well known in many junior sport programs. The letters stand for agility, balance, coordination, speed and strength. Work in the physical skill development of 10u children [11, 12] highlights the development of these skills as essential during this age group. USTA (in common with other sports) has therefore included the development of the ABC'ss as a fundamental part of its 10u programs.

An understanding of each skill highlights the relevance to of all of them to young children in any sport and, because of the age of the players, to 10u tennis in particular. Agility enables a person to move and change direction quickly without a loss of balance. Maintaining balance means that the centre of gravity is over the base of support (the feet in the case of tennis players) and the person can maintain an appropriate body position while moving and/or executing a skill. Balance can be especially difficult for 10u children because of the relative weight of their heads.

Coordination is the 'smooth' linking together of different body segments to produce a skill or a movement. It is usually differentiated into simple, bilateral and complex coordination: the latter is particularly difficult for 10u children. This is because they are increasing their neuromuscular capacities and so are becoming better coordinated, but they often need help.

Speed is concerned both with the rate of movement of individual limbs and also with the rate of movement of the whole body from one place to another. It is a function on physiological development and is therefore a challenge for 10u children.

The last letter in the acronym refers to strength – the energy to move an object against resistance. Tennis requires different types of strength – core, lower and upper body strength – factors that exist at low levels in 10u children, but which improve rapidly in puberty. The maturation of the nervous system in childhood, ahead of the hormonal development associated with muscle development in puberty, is a contributory factor to children becoming stronger. However, it is important that developing strength in 10u children should be undertaken in a different way to that undertaken in puberty. 10u children should be involved in different activities aimed at improving performance that requires strength rather than specific strength and weight-training activities.

These physical/athletic skills are an integral part of the ability of any player to learn sport-specific technical skills and movement. It is generally accepted [11] that their development should be part of any junior sport curriculum, but in a way that meets the *biological age* of the individual. Previous discussion noted the biological age of each child contribute to the specific physical abilities of that child – and thus their technical skills. Here then is another example of where chronological age grouping may impact individual children adversely: either because they are more advanced biologically and so can learn more or different technical skills or because they are biologically behind their chronological age and so need more time on more basic technical skills.

Another consideration in terms of physical/athletic skill development is that 10u boys and girls are physically similar, both in terms of their body shape and also their body fat percentage, so they can learn the same skills in the same way. The differences in the way in which skills can be taught to older boys and girls is therefore not relevant with groups of 10u children: except again when biological age does not match chronological age. In 10u children, the greatest change is in the proportions of the body segments (arms, legs, trunk and head) in relation to each other. 10u children often have agility, balance and coordination challenges, which can be related to the fact that the proportions of the different body segments are changing.

In terms of physical capacities, much research [5, 13] notes differences between 10u children and older children, especially from the onset of puberty. The previous discussion on early onset of puberty with different ethnic groups, however, would indicate that these differences may be apparent in earlier maturing 10u children. Again therefore, the fact that 10u children are in chronological age groups appears problematic in terms of their optimum development.

10u tennis places children of different chronological age on different sizes of court. There are physiological reasons why playing on the correct size of the court is beneficial to any player: distance affects the opportunity to get to the ball and to play longer rallies. The first requires speed and the second requires endurance. As children reach puberty, their anaerobic energy system (which determines their ability to move at speed) matures, enabling them to move quickly for longer and also to 'recognize' when they get tired or hot. Young children have neither the physiological systems that enable them to recognize fatigue, nor the thermoregulation system that enables them to recognize heat or cold. (This means they can become hot or cold more quickly than older children, but without realizing it).

The endurance capacities of 10u children also change as they grow and develop. Limiting factors for the development of endurance are the relative size of the heart, lung volume and the amount of oxygen required for the activity. 10u children have smaller hearts, lower lung volume and a lower ability to take up oxygen from each intake of breath [14]

It can be understood from this discussion that biological age – either earlier or later – impacts the ability of 10u children to develop the different physical capacities and thus a level of skill. This therefore again calls into question the basis of placing 10u players in chronological age groups and on court sizes and in activities that are inappropriate to their biological age.

The Cognitive, Emotional and Social Development of 10u Players

As children get older, their cognitive abilities improve and they become more mature cognitively, emotionally and socially. However, scant real evidence (as against experience) is available in the sport research about psychological skill development in young children and so it is necessary to turn to educational research and the experience of those working with 10u children in contexts other than sports to understand what 10u children can develop/cope with and what age. A number of examples can be given. Cognitively, this age group increasingly understands what they have to do in order to achieve a task. Initially, as 5-year-olds, they copy what they see but have no real understanding of why they are doing something or how to do it. Five and six-year-olds can be taught a few simple rules, while 10-year-olds can also understand the 'unwritten' behavioural rules of the game and learn to respect opponents.

While 6-year-olds find it difficult to even understand winning and losing, 8 and 9-year-olds are learning to cope with the outcomes of both. Five to eight-year-olds believe that if they try hard enough, they will be as good as any other child, but by the age of ten, many children realize that another child is actually more able than them at a particular task. Seven-year-olds find decision-making difficult, but can cope with making choices: to do either this or that. They react to every situation on the tennis court, but ten-year-olds can decide to follow a particular course of action in order to achieve a specific result: they can be proactive. Emotionally, while the 5-year-old needs to achieve every time, the 10-year-old does not need to succeed immediately and can work towards that success. By the age of nine, most children have 'special' friends and can cooperate with, and even help, other children, while 6-year-olds find working with other children more difficult. Five-year-olds will respond to optimal challenges if they think they can do the task, but 10-year-olds usually have enough self-confidence and motivation to take on and try more difficult challenges.

Socially, 5-year-olds find it difficult to work with other children – they are beginning to share, although they still prefer to be the centre of attention.

Mentally, although 5-year-olds cannot listen for long periods, 7-year-olds can follow simple instructions, but are typically unable to concentrate and commit to the same task for very long, while 10-year-olds can focus for a longer period of time and often develop a passion for a particular sport.

Technical and Tactical Development

The development of sport-specific technical and tactical skills in young children is an important part of any junior sport program: the 10u tennis program is simply another example. Malina [15] notes that 'systematic instruction, practise and training are basic to youth development programs and to athlete development'.

In terms of 10u children learning the necessary skills, there are two concepts that affect the ability of each child to make progress in sport and in tennis: trainability and readiness [11, 15]. Trainability links to growth, development and maturation. It considers the individual child's ability (because of his or her stage of growth, development and maturation) to respond to being trained in a specific skill, such as a serve or forehand in tennis. The child may or may not have the necessary physical or athletic skills necessary to perform the activity because of the level of growth, maturity or development. Again, this is the issue of biological and/or developmental age being more appropriate in 10u tennis than chronological age.

Further, the ability of the child will also be affected, in an individual way, by the effectiveness of the teaching of those skills – in other words, if the individual child is ready to learn that skill. It is important to recognize that readiness links both to the ability of the individual child to cope with the environment and to the demands that a specific situation places on that child. Thus, while some children of the same chronological age are physically able to learn a particular skill, other children are not. Further, while a child may be physically able, they may not be 'ready' to learn. Readiness also applies to the competitive environment – a subject to be considered in the next section. In the context of 10u children, it is perfectly possible for a child to be trained in that skill from a physical perspective, but for reasons of readiness, cannot learn it.

Much work has been done on understanding the chronological ages at which specific skills can be taught, assuming the player's readiness to do so. Again, these skills relate to chronological ages of 10u children as a group and so must also be linked to data on the biological and development age of each child.

Competitive Development

Tennis is a game that, for the most part and except in doubles, pits one individual against another. In the context of this chapter, it is the competitive aspect of sport that is particularly affected by the level of cognitive and psychological development of the players. Further, a number of researchers [16–18], parents and coaches are concerned by the impact of competition on 10u children. Bompa [19] noted that 'most young children are not capable of coping with the physical and psychological demands of (high intensity training or) organized competition'.

The principal problem for children is that adult formats (championships, elimination events, rankings and seedings) and concepts (winning, losing, promotion and demotion) of competition are often considered appropriate and necessary for them. In the tennis context, the issue is probably of even greater concern because tennis is an individual sport – without the 'hiding place' that team sports bring.

It was noted above that 10u children have fewer coping skills and we know that they find winning and losing difficult [20]. In tennis, the coping skills do not just relate to winning and losing, but also to umpiring a match while simultaneously playing in it (in other words, making instant and public decisions about balls being in or out). They also relate to dealing with other players and to adult spectators, including coaches and parents.

In 10u tennis (and all junior tennis), a further issue arises: the volume and frequency of competition for 10u children. In reality, some specific issues need to be resolved for 10u tennis: namely the purpose, format and frequency of 10u competition and the impact of competitive stress on 10u players. There needs to be synergy between the purpose of 10u tennis and the needs and abilities of 10u children.

The *purpose* of competition is ill defined in junior tennis as a whole, but especially so for 10u players. At this age, when young children often struggle with the concepts of winning and losing and are learning how to compete, the purpose of competition should be about fun, new experiences and enjoying the process. However, the potential for doing so is limited (especially in an individual sport) when winning and rankings are made so important.

The *format* of competition, given the age of 10u players, is important. The scoring structure was outlined at the beginning of this chapter: it appears to meet the needs of 10u children. However, it is the individual format that is the challenge for many children. In recognizing this, USTA has introduced play days and junior team tennis, but individual competitions still persist from an early age.

So far, this chapter has considered the use of chronological age to decide court sizes and equipment in 10u tennis and the realities of growth and maturation, 'ages' and the physical, psychological, social and competitive development of 10u players. It has noted the possibilities for a lack of synergy. The following section considers the roles and responsibilities of coaches, parents of 10u children and the sport organization (at different levels) for establishing quality systems for 10u children. In doing so, it identifies further issues in the synergistic perspective.

The Role and Responsibilities of Parents, Coaches and the Sport Organization in the 10u Process

Coaches

The vast majority of 10u players begin to learn tennis with a coach, usually in groups, but also in individual lessons. The reasons for the early involvement of a coach are various, but probably include the fact that many parents have not played tennis themselves [21]. In addition, and given that the changes made for 10u tennis are very recent, 100 % of parents will not have learned the game with the 10u equipment themselves! Indeed, in the USA, by the same token, no coach will have learned to play the game with modified equipment – a fact that may explain the initial rejection by many of them to the changes brought about by the 10u program. Further, the training and education of coaches in the rationale and methods of coaching children using modified equipment has only recently gathered momentum. Similarly, the information associated with 10u children's physical, physiological, mental and social development has only recently been considered important and/or relevant. Finally, the research [15] on how children and adults learn skills affects the way in which coaches should coach children especially, but this information has rarely found its way into coach training and education. Thus, for a variety of reasons, perceptible differences exist in the way coaches should coach 10u children now and the way in which they have, until recently, actually done so.

Taking this theme further, coach behaviour and working practise with 10u children or teenagers or adults should be markedly different, simply because each group has very different needs and abilities. Importantly, the coach needs to be able to create an appropriate and different environment [22] for 10u children for the following reasons: It is well known that young children need to have fun, and be with adults whom they like. They need frequent changes of activity to match their rapidly changing attention levels. They learn principally by copying. They want to be with their friends, even if their friends are better or worse then themselves. Coaches therefore need to create a fun, non-threatening environment, have a range and variety of ideas and use visual stimuli (demonstrations and activities). They need to teach children to be active and reduce the amount of verbal information that they give. For many coaches, and especially those who have been trained in methods more suitable to working with older children and adults, creating such an environment where children also learn skills through play and trial and error can be challenging or even impossible. Many coaches still put children in lines so that they can be 'fed' perfect balls to hit. Children want to move, and tennis is a game of movement and using a variety of different skills in a random way. Standing in lines is neither relevant nor enjoyable to a 10u child. Additionally, learning to play in an environment that is not related to the game is not fun for 10u children. Finally, coaches new to 10u tennis are often unaware of the impact of growth, maturation and development. They expect 10u players to be as physically, technically and cognitively able as older children and teenagers.

They find it difficult to scale what they teach to fit the needs and abilities of 10u children.

On a similar note, coaches often presume that 10u children enjoy and can cope with adult forms of tennis competition, i.e. individual matches in tournaments, with a strong emphasis on winning, probably because they were competitive players themselves. In reality, 10u players need more team events where the emphasis is on fun and learning how to compete with their friends and not against children they do not know.

Finally, but importantly, in terms of coaching knowledge is the need for coaches to know how to organize and develop programs, lesson content and lesson frequency that are appropriate for 10u children. Research [11, 19] recommends that the volume of physical activity undertaken by 10u children should be proportionally less than it is for older children and adults. Further, research also shows that [11, 23] young children should play a variety of different sports and activities because doing so will give them a wider range of physical skills and experiences. Yet, and in contrast, by the age of 8 or 9, some children will develop a preference for a particular sport and may be showing an aptitude for one in particular. In tennis terms, experience indicates that the modified equipment does help many children develop higher quality skills at a younger age and become 'successful' [2]. Conversely, experience also indicates that coaches (and in some instances, the organization) encourage increased training and competition for such a child as a result of early success. Coaches (and as will be discussed later), parents and the sport organization should be very aware of the possible outcomes of increasing the tennis and competition volume and frequency for a young player. Experience shows the point where a 10u child is, at best, playing and competing too much, or at worst, is 'specializing' early in the sport, can be reached quite quickly. Early specialization indicates that the child focuses on one sport all year round [24, 25]. It is linked to the early junior (but rarely adult) success that often comes at a cost to the young athlete in terms of negative social, emotional and physical outcomes and even injury.

This discussion on coaches indicates that a further lack of synergy can exist between the individual needs of 10u children and the coaching they receive. The suggestion can be made that coach training and education in the changed 10u tennis environment has lagged behind the use of modified equipment: a fact that can lead to coach behaviour and a low level of knowledge and skills that does not match the needs of 10u children.

Parents

Earlier in the chapter, a lack of tennis 'experience' by many parents [21] was noted. Perhaps too, parents assume that coaches and the sport organization will deliver the appropriate tennis product. For certain, the vast majority of parents want only the best for their child and will trust coaches and the sport organization to deliver the 'correct' product for the age of their child. As this chapter makes evident however, on occasions, a lack of synergy exists between the needs and abilities of an individual child and the programs. At this point, parents who know their child can become concerned [21], but even then assume that the coach and the tennis organization know best and so run with them. A familiar situation in many 10u programs is that a child is moved to the next court size and ball and racquet for reasons other than growth and development. Frequently, the child then is playing without their friends and can lose confidence because of a lack of continued success. Of similar concern, and referred to previously, as children improve, they may be encouraged to have more lessons, enter more competitions and quickly specialise in tennis. Parents are often uninformed regarding the benefits of the appropriate use of courts and equipment at 10u level and so may not understand best practise.

The Sport Organization

Typically, in any sport, the organizational structure can exist at different levels: international, national, regional, city and club. At the beginning of this chapter, the ITF was noted to be the international proponent of 10u tennis, with different tennis federations including USTA, taking responsibility for 10u tennis at the national level. However, within a nation, the organization of the sport varies from sport to sport. USTA has sections (regions), states, districts and clubs: each has the ability to frame elements of the 10u tennis program as it wishes, but (hopefully) using USTA guidelines. The key organizational issues of concern from the perspective of synergy in 10u tennis in the USA are the designated court sizes and equipment by chronological age, the training and education of coaches and the competitive structure for 10u children. Chronological age and coach training and education is the responsibility of USTA. Both have been discussed previously and the issues highlighted.

However, to a large extent, 10u competitive structures are initiated at district, state and sectional level and not specifically by USTA itself until very recently. It appears that best practise in terms of 10u competitive structures is difficult to achieve when responsibilities are distributed to lower levels of the organization, possibly because other and/or more local factors add to the challenge of doing what is best for 10u children. Reference has already been made to the fact that the advent of 10u tennis is recent with a consequent lack of experience of it for many coaches and also adult players – and, by default, organizers. 10u tournaments are run by sections or states and are frequently elimination events with only one winner: a fact that could be attributed to the lack of adult experience of 10u players or competitive options. The festival type approach where children learn to be competitors and have fun, play in teams in non-elimination events [26] is largely absent, except where initiated by USTA. Instead, rankings (a feature of adult tennis) are commonly used in 10u tennis. As a consequence, a system has been created that satisfies an apparent adult need. Further, and significantly, the system is designed to move children to the next court and ball on the basis of their results, irrespective of their age, skills or size and seemingly as quickly as possible. A phenomenon known as the 'race to the yellow ball' has been created across the USA that is at variance even with the national policy of chronological age for specific courts and equipment.

The Need for Synergy

The thesis that has been presented in this chapter is that a lack of synergy between objectives and processes in 10u tennis exists and actually, in competitive terms, contradicts national policy. Synergy in 10u tennis, if properly implemented, would present opportunities for children to gain high levels of skill on the appropriate court and with the right equipment for them as an individual. At the same time, both of USTA's objectives could to be realized. Each young player would learn to play and also compete in an environment appropriate to his or her needs and abilities and not the chronological age. Such a principle of alignment would, de facto, recognize the needs of individual children who, by the very fact that they are growing and maturing, are dissimilar to other children of the same chronological age. Using the correct court sizes and equipment for the individual would help each child develop the specific physical, technical and movement skills that are possible at his or her 'age' and stage.

Competitive systems would be created that used appropriate formats, scoring and length of matches for the stage and purpose of competitive development at each stage. At present, there is very little evidence to suggest that the use of rankings in 10u tennis is a concern because excellence has become the only criterion and is used to 'progress' a child to the next court. Further, the use of ratings, developed specifically for 10u players would enable children to play against others of a similar standard, has seemingly not been considered. In 2009, the UK Coaching Framework noted the imperative of making sure that the needs and abilities of every child were at the heart of each system and the focus was not solely on structures that catered for excellence [27].

All of these examples and those cited throughout the chapter have highlighted elements that need to be considered in 10u tennis systems and programs: for example, different ages, stages of growth and social development. There is an additional consideration: the principle that each part of a 10u programs should align with every other part: for example, competitive structures should line up with the mental, emotional and social needs of 10u children. At present, they do not do so. How an individual child who is 'at variance' to the norms for his or her chronological age is catered for is important to the successful tennis development of that child. At present, the necessary synergy for that to happen does not appear to exist.

10u tennis should be thought of as one step in the long-term development of the child as a tennis player. Often, the fact that Bompa's [19] notion that a 'gradual, progressive program with no abrupt increases in intensities greatly increases training efficiency and reduces the chance of frustration and injury' is ignored. Moving a child to the next court size or ball simply because they have won a few matches thus ignores Bompa's thesis. Of further concern is that the use of incorrect equipment and the probable increase in practise and competition adds to the potential for injury of both a physical and mental/emotional/social nature. It decreases the chances of effective long-term development and thus more participants and future world-class players.

10u tennis has the potential to achieve the twin objectives of USTA and those of any other nation provided that synergy can be established between group and individual needs and abilities, coach training and education and 10u competitive structures.

References

1. Elliott BC, Reid MM, Crespo M. Technique development in tennis stroke production. London: International Tennis Federation; 2009.
2. Farrow D, Reid M. The effect of equipment scaling on the skill acquisition of beginning tennis players. J Sports Sci. 2010;28(7):723–32. doi:10.1080/02640411003770238.
3. Larson EJ, Guggenheimer JD. The effects of scaling tennis equipment on the forehand ground-stroke performance of children. J Sports Sci Med. 2013;12(2):323–31.
4. Beunen G, Malina R. Growth and biologic maturation: relevance to athletic performance. In: Hebestreit H, Bar-Or O. editors. The young athlete. The encyclopaedia of sports medicine X111. Malden: Blackwell Publishing; 2008. p. 3–17
5. Malina RM, Bouchard C, Bar-Or O. Growth, maturation and physical activity. Champaign, IL: Human Kinetics; 2004.
6. Welsman JR, Armstrong N. Interpreting performance in relation to body size. In: Armstrong N, editor. Paediatric exercise physiology. Edinburgh: Elsevier; 2007. p. 27–46.
7. Herman-Giddens ME, Steffes J, Harris D, Slora E, Hussey M, Dowshen SA, Reiter EO. Secondary sexual characteristics in boys: data from the pediatric research in office settings network. Pediatrics. 2012;130(5):1058–68. doi:10.1542/peds.2011-3291.
8. Baxter- Jones ADG, Sherar LB. Growth and maturation. In: Armstrong N, editor. Paediatric exercise physiology. Edinburgh: Elsevier; 2007. p. 1–26.
9. Lloyd RS, Oliver JL. Strength and conditioning of young athletes: science and application. London: Routledge; 2014.
10. Cobley S, Wattie N, Baker J, McKenna J. Annual age-grouping and athlete development: a meta-analytical review of relative age effects in sport. Sports Med. 2009;39(3):235–56.
11. Balyi I, Way R, Higgs C. Long-term athlete development. Leeds: Human Kinetics; 2013.
12. Foreman G, Bradshaw A. An introduction to the FUNdamentals of movement. Leeds: 1st4Sport.com; 2009.
13. Rowland TW. Developmental exercise physiology. Champaign: Human Kinetics; 1996.
14. Winsley RJ. Cardiovascular function. In: Armstrong N, editor. Paediatric exercise physiology. Edinburgh: Elsevier; 2007. p. 139–60.
15. Malina RM. Skill acquisition in childhood and adolescence. In: Hebestreit H, Bar-Or O, editors. The young athlete. The encyclopaedia of sports medicine X111. Malden: Blackwell Publishing; 2008. p. 96–111.
16. Baxter-Jones ADG. Growth and development of young athletes – should competition levels be age related? Sports Med. 1995;20(2):59–64.
17. Bloom B. Developing talent in young people. New York: Ballantine Books; 1985.
18. Côté J. The influence of the family in the development of talent in sport. Sports Psychol. 1999;13(4):395–417.
19. Bompa TO. Total training for young champions. Champaign: Human Kinetics; 2000.

20. Gould D, Dieffenbach K. Psychological characteristics and their development in Olympic champions. J Appl Sport Psychol. 2002;14(3):172–204.
21. Pankhurst A, Collins D. Talent identification and development in junior performance tennis: a strategy to support the parent role (in review).
22. Vickers JN. Skill acquisition: designing optimal learning environments. In: Collins D, Button A, Richards H, editors. Performance psychology: a practitioner's guide. Oxford: Churchill Livingstone; 2008. p. 191–206.
23. Côté J, Baker J, Abernethy B. Play and practice in the development of sport expertise. In: Tenenbaum G, Eklund RC, editors. Handbook of sport psychology. New York: Wiley; 2007. p. 184–202.
24. American Academy of Pediatrics Committee on Sports Medicine and Fitness. Intensive training and sports specialization in young athletes. Pediatrics. 2000;106(1):154–7.
25. National Association for Sport and Physical Education. Guidelines for participation in youth sport programs: specialisation versus multi-sport participation [Position statement]. Reston: 2010.
26. International Tennis Federation. 10 and under tennis a guide for tennis parents. www.playandstay.com/tennis10s/overview.aspx.
27. North J. The coaching workforce 2009–2016. Leeds: Sports Coach UK; 2009.

Chapter 2
Growth and Development in the Young Athlete

Sarah E. Strandjord and Ellen S. Rome

Stages of Adolescence

There are three general stages of adolescence—early, middle, and late—distinguished by common physical, cognitive, and psychosocial changes. Table 2.1 outlines various facets of early, middle, and late stages of development. Rate of progression through these facets varies among individuals but generally follows a predictable pattern. This developmental sequence is shaped both by biological factors, particularly hormonal changes, and psychosocial factors, particularly support from parents, peers, and other role models. Understanding the typical progression from childhood to adulthood is essential for promoting healthy physical and mental growth among young athletes.

Physical Development

Puberty, a biological process primarily governed by hormonal changes, marks the beginning of adolescence and the progression to reproductive maturity. The process of sexual maturation is governed by two hormonal axes—the

S.E. Strandjord, BS
Cleveland Clinic Lerner College of Medicine of Case Western University,
Cleveland, OH, USA
e-mail: strands@ccf.org

E.S. Rome, MD, MPH (✉)
Center for Adolescent Medicine, Cleveland Clinic, Cleveland, OH, USA

Department of General Pediatrics, Cleveland Clinic Children's Hospital,
Cleveland, OH, USA
e-mail: romee@ccf.org

© Springer International Publishing Switzerland 2016
A.C. Colvin, J.N. Gladstone (eds.), *The Young Tennis Player: Injury Prevention and Treatment,* Contemporary Pediatric and Adolescent Sports Medicine,
DOI 10.1007/978-3-319-27559-8_2

Table 2.1 Characteristics of early, middle, and late adolescence [1]

	Early (11–14 years)	Middle (15–17 years)	Late (18–21 years)
Central question	Am I normal?	Am I liked?	Am I loved?
Physical	Onset of puberty Growth acceleration	Continued sexual development (maturation in most girls) Continued growth	Sexual maturity Slowed growth
Cognitive	Concrete thinking	Emerging abstract thinking Emotion-driven behavior	Formalized abstract thinking Future-driven behavior
Self-perception	Self-conscious about appearance	Exploration of different personas	More stable self-identity
Family relationships	Increased need for privacy	Peak of parental conflict	Independence from family
Peers relationships	Same-sex peer groups	Mixed-sex peer groups Dating relationships	One-on-one relationships

hypothalamic-pituitary-adrenal axis and the hypothalamic-pituitary-gonadal axis (Fig. 2.1). The adrenal axis is typically activated first, resulting in a rise in androgen production. This rise may occur as early as 6 years of age and is sometimes associated with body odor and, in a small number of children, premature adrenarche or the appearance of sexual hair in girls younger than 8 years of age or boys younger than 9 years of age [2]. The true onset of puberty, however, coincides with activation of the gonadal axis. A rise in pulsatile gonadotropin-releasing hormone (GnRH) secretion from the hypothalamus stimulates secretion of luteinizing hormone (LH) and follicle-stimulating hormone (FSH) from the anterior pituitary. LH and FSH then stimulate gonadal production and secretion of androgens and, in females, estrogens.

Female Sexual Maturation

In the United States, girls usually begin puberty earlier than boys, with the typical onset of breast development, or thelarche, between the ages of 8 and 12 years. Thelarche, which is primarily under the control of estrogens secreted by the ovaries, is divided into five developmental stages described by the Tanner scale (Fig. 2.2a). Tanner 1 is prepubertal. Tanner 2 indicates the start of thelarche with the formation of a breast bud localized to the nipple. In Tanner 3, the breast bud extends beyond the nipple and areola (the darker pigmented area around the nipple). In Tanner 4, the areola becomes a separate mound on top of the primary mound of the developing breast. Tanner 5, the adult breast, is achieved when the areola becomes flush with the breast with a protruding nipple. In normal boys ages 11–15 years, breast buds may develop and then regress by age 14–16 years. Progression to Tanner 3 breasts in a male, however, indicates gynecomastia and deserves attention from a pediatrician or endocrinologist.

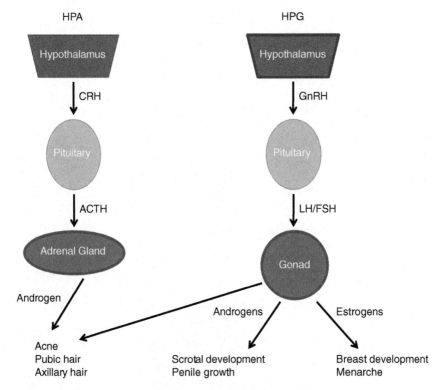

Fig. 2.1 Regulation of hormonal changes during puberty by the hypothalamic-pituitary-adrenal (*HPA*) axis and the hypothalamic-pituitary-gonadal (*HPG*) axis

Pubic hair development (Fig. 2.2b), called adrenarche, generally progresses along with breast development. However, because pubic hair development is predominantly controlled by androgens secreted by the adrenal glands, the two developmental processes are not always simultaneous. Adrenarche follows a similar trajectory for girls and boys. Tanner 1 is prepubertal with no pubic hair. Tanner 2 occurs with the first appearance of downy hair (easily countable). In Tanner 3, hair becomes more coarse and curly and extends laterally into an upside-down triangle (countable only if obsessive compulsive). In Tanner 4, hair extends across pubis and forms a more dense upside-down triangle (too many to count) and, by Tanner 5, extends to the thighs. A majority but not all adolescents progress to Tanner 4 or 5 pubic hair.

Menarche, the onset of menstruation, occurs about 2 years following the onset of female puberty, usually between the ages of 10–14 years. The timing of puberty is not completely understood but appears to be influenced by genetic as well as environmental factors, including adiposity, nutrition, physical activity, and exposure to endocrine-disrupting chemicals [4, 5]. Changes in these factors, such as the rise in obesity in developed countries, are thought to contribute to the decreasing age of menarche observed over the past few decades [6, 7].

Fig. 2.2 Tanner stages of sexual maturity in girls. (**a**) Tanner stages of breast development. *Stage 1*, preadolescent; *stage 2*, breast bud forms with elevation of areola and papilla; *stage 3*, enlargement of breast and areola; *stage 4*, projection of areola to form a secondary mound above the level of the breast; and *stage 5*, areola returns to the general contour of the breast. (**b**) Tanner stages of pubic hair development in girls. *Stage 2*, sparse downy hair chiefly on labia (base of penis for boys); *stage 3*, hair extends laterally and becomes more coarse and curly; *stage 4*, adult-like hair extending across pubis but sparing thighs; and *stage 5*, hair extends to medial thighs (Reprinted with permission from [3])

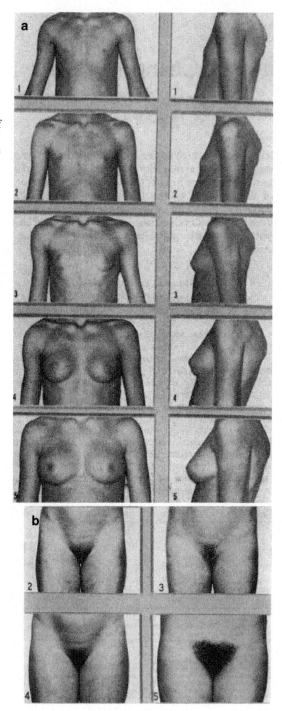

Male Sexual Maturation

In males, puberty begins with an increase in testicular volume between the ages of 9 and 14 years (Fig. 2.3). Tanner 1, prepubertal, progresses to Tanner 2 with scrotal enlargement and thinning of the scrotal skin. Tanner 3 is marked by initial penile growth, primarily in length, and further scrotal enlargement. In Tanner 4, the penis grows in girth as well as length and the scrotal skin darkens. By Tanner 5, the genitals have reached their adult size and appearance. Pubic hair develops as described in the previous section on female puberty (Fig. 2.2b). In males, pubic hair growth is closely correlated to the growth of the penis since both processes are governed by androgens. Discordance between these two sequences can occur with some disease conditions that affect the adrenal glands or testicles and therefore deserves medical attention.

Growth Acceleration

Growth acceleration begins in early adolescence for both girls and boys but reaches its peak velocity, known as the "growth spurt", at different times depending on gender. In girls, the peak height velocity typically occurs during Tanner stage 2 (Fig. 2.4). The peak height velocity in girls is about 8.3 cm/year. Boys, in contrast, reach their peak height velocity around the time of Tanner stage 4, 2–3 years later than girls, and reach a higher velocity of about 9.5 cm/year (Fig. 2.4). This

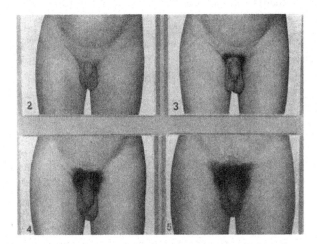

Fig. 2.3 Tanner stages in gonadal and pubic hair development in boys. *Stage 2*, enlargement of testes and scrotum with thinning and reddening of scrotal skin; *stage 3*, enlargement of penis in length and further enlargement of scrotum; *stage 4*, enlargement of penis in length and circumference and further enlargement scrotum with darkening of scrotal skin; and *stage 5*, adult genitalia (Reprinted with permission from [8])

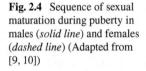

Fig. 2.4 Sequence of sexual maturation during puberty in males (*solid line*) and females (*dashed line*) (Adapted from [9, 10])

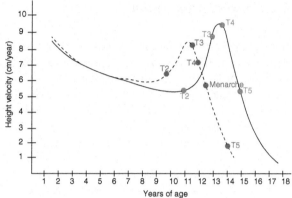

difference in velocity and timing eventually results in higher stature in males compared to females.

The sequence of musculoskeletal growth creates a vulnerable period of reduced balance, flexibility, and bone strength. Growth acceleration occurs first in the distal limbs followed by the proximal limbs and, in late adolescence, the trunk [11]. This asynchronous growth pattern results in long limbs with little axial support, leading to a decline in balance and coordination during early and middle adolescence. In addition, because bone growth outpaces the growth of muscle and tendons, adolescent joints have reduced flexibility. As bone grows, it initially forms a matrix that is later mineralized to improve strength and rigidity. In adolescents, bone mineralization lags behind matrix formation by up to a year, resulting in a period where the new bone is soft and more prone to fracture [12, 13]. Thus, especially during peak height velocity, adolescents have an increased risk of strains, sprains, and fractures.

Coaching the Developing Body: Preventing Injury During Growth

Sports are the main cause of injury in adolescents. As described above, adolescence is a period of particular risk of injury due to the rate and sequence of musculoskeletal growth. Injury can have both short-term and long-term consequences, including economic costs, inability to participate in sporting activity, and early osteoarthritis [14]. Nearly two million US adolescents go to the emergency department each year for injuries related to sports or recreation activities [15]. In adolescent tennis players, ankle sprains are the most frequent cause of acute injury, followed by knee injuries such as anterior cruciate ligament (ACL) tears [16]. Chronic overuse injuries, including lateral epicondylitis (i.e., "tennis elbow"), shoulder pain, back pain, and metacarpal stress fractures, are also common in young tennis players [16–19].

Preventing injuries relies on having sport programs that emphasize proper technique, conditioning, rest, and psychological health. Research on preventive strategies in adolescent sports has shown that preseason and in-season conditioning programs have the potential to decrease the risk of injury. The most effective programs are those that include strength, flexibility, balance, and sport-specific technique training [14]. Adequate rest, particularly following an injury, is also important to avoid overuse injury and long-term damage. Current recommendations are that young athletes take off 1–2 days a week and 2–3 months a year from their sport [20]. In addition, incorporating strategies to combat the emotional and psychological stress of sport participation can help to protect adolescents from overtraining and burnout, as discussed in later sections.

Cognitive Development

Adolescence is a period of rapid change in brain structure and function. During this period, more complex thinking processes emerge as adolescents transition from concrete thinking (i.e., thinking focused on actual objects and experiences) to abstract thinking (i.e., thinking characterized by the use of concepts and generalizations). This transition leads to improved judgment, risk assessment, emotional regulation, and self-direction. In addition to improvements in reasoning, adolescents also exhibit improvements in information processing, particularly processing efficiency and capacity, and improvements in visuospatial control of movement.

Executive Function

Cognitive changes in adolescents are largely attributed to the development of brain regions involved in executive function, particularly the prefrontal cortex [21]. The prefrontal cortex is essential for planning, decision-making, and regulating social behavior. Numerous studies in cognitive behavioral research have demonstrated better performance on tasks that involve the dorsolateral prefrontal cortex, a region involved in working memory and planning, and the ventromedial prefrontal cortex, a region involved in evaluating risk and reward, in adolescents compared to children [22–24]. These behavioral studies are further corroborated by neurostructural studies that have shown increased growth and improved connectivity in these regions throughout adolescence [25]. The effects of these changes can also be observed in the sport environment. During middle adolescence, for example, young tennis players may be able to study their opponent and think through strategies that would utilize their own strengths while minimizing those of their opponent. This process involves abstract thought (the ability to apply knowledge to hypothetical situations) as well as executive function (the ability to plan and execute a game strategy). As described in the next section, however, these newfound skills are typically not applied to all realms of thought or action until late adolescence.

Risk Seeking

Despite evidence of development within brain regions associated with executive function, adolescents continue to exhibit impulsive and irrational behavior well into middle adolescence. This apparent paradox is explained by a theory that, while the brain is rapidly developing, it continues to be immature [26]. Therefore, like a toddler who is cognitively ready to walk but lacks coordination due to inexperience, a teenager may be cognitively ready to regulate his or her behavior but lacks coordination to effectively use those skills. In addition, research suggests that subcortical regions of the brain involved in emotion and reward, particularly the amygdala and the nucleus accumbens, mature earlier than the prefrontal cortex [25, 27]. This mismatch in brain development leads to increased risk-taking and sensation-seeking behavior during adolescence (Fig. 2.5). While both sexes follow this general pattern of development, female adolescents generally exhibit lower risk-taking behavior and higher impulse control compared to males and, similar to pubertal development, reach peak levels of risk taking earlier than males [28].

Continuing the example from the previous section, while middle adolescents may be able to develop strategies to succeed in their next match, they may not have the foresight to avoid distractions the night before a match that will interfere with their performance. The immediate satisfaction from staying up late to text friends, browse the internet, or watch TV often overrides the decision to sleep in order to perform better tomorrow. Strategies to oppose these drives might include setting time limits on distracting behaviors or setting aside designated time for these distractions. On a more serious level, some adolescents may also choose to drink alcohol or do drugs for the immediate gratification they receive from their peers and the substance itself. They often understand the risks, including expulsion from the team or physical harm, but adhere to the "it won't happen to me" mindset. Minimizing this type of risk-taking behavior requires limiting

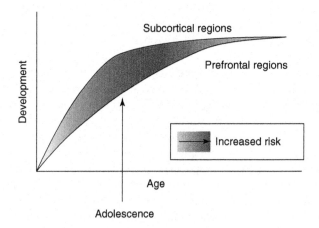

Fig. 2.5 Model representing the different rates in maturation of the subcortical and prefrontal regions of the brain. The size of the gap (*shaded*) in maturity between these regions correlates with increased risk of emotionally driven behavior (Reprinted with permission from [27])

access to adverse influences and improving access to safe environments, such as organized sport activities or clubs through the school or community.

Visuospatial Processing

Changes in the parietal lobe, which is responsible for integrating auditory, visual, and tactile signals, are also observed during adolescence. The parietal lobe combines sensory information, such as the shape of an object, its relation to surrounding structures, and body position, to create a visuospatial map and coordinate a motor response. Brain remodeling in the parietal lobe typically peaks in middle adolescence with earlier development in girls than in boys. This development is essential for improving visuospatial control of movement during sports and helps to explain the improvements in coordination seen in older adolescent athletes. In tennis, for example, parietal function allows a player to adapt his or her body and racket movement to different circumstances, resulting in a more accurate stroke. Adolescence is therefore an ideal time to refine motor skills and control in young athletes.

Coaching the Developing Brain: Adapting to Different Abilities

Rates of brain development can vary widely among individuals, with variations both in global cognition and in specific brain regions. In the athletic setting, it is important to assess the cognitive stage of individual athletes and to adapt coaching methods accordingly. Younger adolescents, for example, may have difficulty accurately performing complex movements or planning hypothetical strategies for an upcoming match. An effective coach will recognize these limitations to avoid frustration while continuing to build on the athlete's current skill set. In addition, anticipating potential challenges, such as impulsive behaviors or emotional volatility during matches, can help to reduce adverse effects on individual and team morale. Coaches should, for example, set clear guidelines for behavior and consequences for violating those guidelines. Participation in sports provides opportunities for teens to further develop their cognitive abilities, both by improving physical and mental coordination and by practicing group cooperation. Coaches hold the unique position to create an environment that accepts individual variations in ability and promotes good choices both on and off the court.

Psychosocial Development

Adolescence is characterized by significant changes in social relationships as teens attempt to establish identities that are independent from their parents and family. During the typical progression of psychosocial development, adolescents shift their focus from more superficial concerns of external appearance and peer acceptance to more reflective questions about who they are, who they want to become, and who they want to spend their lives with. This process often involves changes in self-expression, inner turmoil, and risky experimentation that can strain relationships with parents and other family members.

Self-Perception

Early adolescence is typically plagued by self-consciousness in response to the physical changes of puberty. During this stage of development, individuals are often preoccupied with external appearance, constantly comparing their bodies to those of their peers and those portrayed in the media. Young adolescents may also experience a "personal fable" in which they believe that they are the focus of everyone else's attention, adding to their feelings of both uniqueness and self-consciousness. As teens progress into middle adolescence, they often become more accepting of their changing bodies and, as a result, start to experiment with different personas. Frequent changes in styles of dress, friend groups, and interests are common during this stage as adolescents start to ask the question, "Who am I?" In late adolescence, as physical changes slow down, individuals develop a more stable body image and self-identity. Older adolescents begin to think more independently and typically become less self-centered.

Coaching the Developing Mind: Detecting Body Image Dissatisfaction

Young athletes, like all adolescents, experience challenges with body image. In females, this body distress can manifest as a syndrome referred to as "the female athlete triad"—disordered eating, menstrual dysfunction, and decreased bone mineral density. At least one component of the triad is present in up to three-fourths of female adolescent athletes [29]. This triad is most common in sports that emphasize low body weight, such as long-distance running, gymnastics, figure skating, and dancing. Other sports, including tennis, have also been associated with an increased risk of different components of the female athlete triad, particularly disordered eating and menstrual irregularities [30]. Recently, the 2014 International Olympic committee introduced a new term, "Relative Energy Deficiency in Sport" (RED-S), to encompass those athletes who do not fully meet the criteria for the female athlete triad, including males, but may still experience its consequences [31, 32]. Relative energy deficiency is defined as energy expenditure that outweighs energy intake, which can have adverse effects on nearly every body system, including the reproductive, musculoskeletal, cardiovascular, and immune systems. Athletes are at increased risk of relative energy deficiency because of increased caloric requirements from regular strenuous activity and increased pressure to maintain a particular physique.

Prevention of RED-S and the female athlete triad requires early detection of warning signs, including weight loss, mood changes, dissatisfaction with appearance, decline in performance, and frequent illness, injury, or fractures. Energy repletion is the cornerstone of treatment along with multidisciplinary support from physicians, dietitians, mental health professionals, coaches, and family members [33]. Young athletes exhibiting warning signs should be referred to a health-care professional with experience in disordered eating as soon as possible. Early recognition is essential to prevent irreversible effects on physical and psychological health, growth, and sport performance.

Social Relationships in Early Adolescence

The transition from childhood to adulthood involves a gradual separation, both emotionally and economically, from parents and the family. This process begins in early adolescence with the formation of primarily same-sex peer groups [34]. These peer groups are often idealized and strongly influence how adolescents express themselves, such as through clothing, language, and activities, to fit in with the group (Fig. 2.6a). During this period, adolescents will often have an increased desire for privacy, a decreased interest in family activities, and a blatant disregard for parental advice regarding behavior or appearance. As a result of this separation, adolescents may seek role models outside of the family, such as through coaches, personal trainers, or older athletes. Sport participation can therefore provide a sense of belonging without disrupting the natural drive for autonomy.

Social Relationships in Middle Adolescence

In middle adolescence, peer relationships gain increasing importance as adolescents become involved in mixed-sex peer groups and seek further independence from the family (Fig. 2.6b) [34]. Dating often begins at this stage, usually with short relationships characterized by intense emotion, physical attraction, and sexual experimentation. Middle adolescence is also when many youth acknowledge their sexual identity and orientation. This time of development is often the peak of teen-parental conflict. It is also a particularly sensitive period for the development of anxiety, depression, and loneliness as a result of perceived rejection by peers, potential romantic partners, and particularly in adolescents with same-sex attractions, family members [35, 36]. These stressors can impact athletic performance and concentration.

Social Relationships in Late Adolescence

By late adolescence, most adolescents have established a separate identity from their parents. They begin to place less importance on the peer group and more importance on intimate one-on-one relationships (Fig. 2.6c) [34]. These

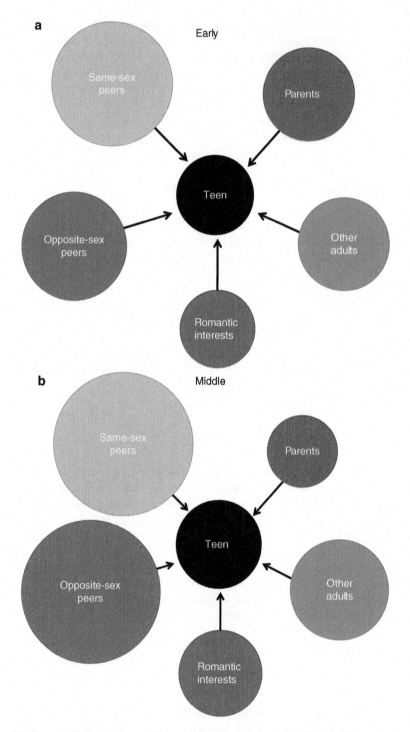

Fig. 2.6 Degree of influence from different social groups during (**a**) early, (**b**) middle, and (**c**) late adolescence

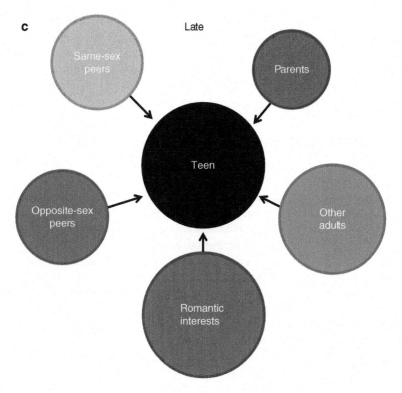

Fig. 2.6 (continued)

relationships tend to be less superficial than those of middle adolescence with more emphasis on intimacy and increasing commitment. In preparation for adulthood, late adolescence is also a period when individuals often make career goals and future plans for their role in society. This shifting perspective correlates with the development of more mature thinking processes along with a firmer self-identity, allowing late adolescents to apply their values and goals to future ambitions.

Coaching the Developing Individual: Supporting Athlete Autonomy

Social development during adolescence involves an increasing need for both acceptance and independence. Sports provide an opportunity for young athletes to interact with peers who share a common interest, often creating a sense of belonging. In addition, mentoring relationships between coaches and athletes can help compensate for the guidance adolescents no longer seek from their parents. Coaches can also make sport training a chance for adolescents to exercise their autonomy in a safe environment. Studies show that supporting independence in sports is an effective way to improve self-esteem, maintain intrinsic motivation, and decrease dropout

[37, 38]. Multiple tactics can be used to create a climate that promotes autonomy, including providing choices for practice activities or match strategies, offering rationales for planned activities, acknowledging athletes' feelings and perspectives, and providing constructive feedback [39]. This approach allows adolescents to take responsibility for their own development both as athletes and as individuals.

Parental Role in Young Athlete Development

Adolescence is a transitional period for parents as well as their children. Parents no longer experience the same level of companionship or maintain the same level of authority they had during earlier stages of childhood. Navigating this new role requires parents to let go of their old relationship and, gradually, their child as he or she experiments with independence. For the parents of young athletes, this process involves finding ways to support adolescents in their sport without attempting to control their performance. Sports can be a healthy venue for adolescent growth and development, but the greatest benefit comes when young athletes participate on their own accord and set their own goals. Parents play an important role by providing appropriate encouragement while helping athletes navigate the challenges of sport participation, such as failures and stress.

Support Without Pressure

There is a fine line between creating an environment of support and creating an environment of pressure. Studies looking at how young athletes view parental participation in sports consistently show that players want their parents to be involved in their sport [40–42]. Players who perceive pressure from their parents to perform, however, tend to have less motivation and less enjoyment [40]. A study in young tennis players found that athletes preferred their parents to provide comments on non-tactical aspects of performance, such as attitude and effort, rather than critiquing their performance and attempting to coach [42]. As part of the adolescent drive for independence, young athletes generally prefer parents to take on an observational role in their sport. Being overly controlling can discourage participation by making the court an extension of the home rather than a place for teens to find structure and support outside the family.

Achievement by Proxy

One of the dangers of parental over-involvement is "achievement by proxy." This phrase describes a condition where a parent or other involved adult lives vicariously through the accomplishments of his or her child. As a result, the underlying motivation for sports participation is skewed toward the goals of the adult rather than those of the athlete. This skewed perspective of success leads not only to excess pressure on the teen but also, potentially, to neglect and abuse as parental ambitions take precedence over the desires, needs, and health of the child [43]. It is therefore crucial that parents monitor their motivations by asking, "Am I doing this for my child or for myself?"[44] Supporting a young athlete requires maintaining realistic expectations based on his or her stage of development as well as regularly reassessing the goals of sport participation for the child, the parent, the coach, and other involved individuals. Parents and coaches should work together to provide a positive sport experience that matches the desires and physical abilities of the athlete.

Preventing Burnout

Burnout—physical or emotional exhaustion leading to decreased sport enjoyment and accomplishment—is a common problem among young athletes [45]. The condition is considered a response to chronic physical and psychological stress. Risk factors include both environmental factors, such as high time demands and high performance expectations, and personality traits, such as perfectionism, low self-esteem, and high anxiety. Stress reduction techniques lie at the center of both prevention and treatment of burnout. Daily tools, such as deep breathing or reciting affirmations (Box 2.1), can help athletes to relax and maintain a positive attitude [46]. In addition, taking regular breaks from their sport will allow adolescents to rest their bodies and avoid overuse injuries. Current recommendations are that adolescents take off 1–2 days per week from organized sports and 2–3 months a year from training and competition [20]. Lastly, it is essential that both parents and coaches maintain reasonable expectations based on the physical, cognitive, and psychosocial stage of an athlete.

Box 2.1. Helpful Affirmations for Young Athletes
- I let any stress just flow over or past me, without absorbing it into my body.
- I can do my work quickly and well, while staying physically relaxed.
- I am able to deal well with stress, extra work, or excitement, without triggering any uncomfortable symptoms.
- I have the power to choose how I respond to everything in my life.
- I handle any problems with a calm mind and relaxed body.
- I am able to change anything in my life.
- All my old habits and thoughts are just memories. I can replace them at any time with new habits of positive thoughts and peacefulness.

Reprinted with permission from [46]

Conclusion

Adolescence is a period of change and passage. Supporting young athletes as they transition from childhood to adulthood requires a delicate balance of providing guidance and permitting independence. As their bodies grow, adolescents must learn to adapt their motor skills in order to take into account new abilities as well as new limitations. As their brains develop, they must learn to practice behavioral control and consider other perspectives in order to achieve personal goals and function as a team. As their social relationships shift, they must learn to find support from outside the family in order to establish their own individual identities. Sport participation can have a positive impact on each aspect of adolescent development by providing young athletes with a safe environment to express and challenge themselves. At the same time, however, working with young athletes comes with unique challenges, including increased risk of injury, rebellious behavior, emotional volatility, and a growing desire for independence. Successfully navigating these challenges requires understanding and support from family members, coaches, and other figures involved in the adolescent's life.

References

1. Rome E. The adolescent. In: Lang R, Hensrud D, editors. Clinical preventive medicine. 2nd ed. Chicago: American Medical Association Press; 2004. p. 290–300.
2. Auchus RJ, Rainey WE. Adrenarche – physiology, biochemistry and human disease. Clin Endocrinol (Oxf). 2004;60(3):288–96.
3. Marshall WA, Tanner JM. Variations in pattern of pubertal changes in girls. Arch Dis Child. 1969;44(235):291–303.
4. Euling SY, Selevan SG, Pescovitz OH, Skakkebaek NE. Role of environmental factors in the timing of puberty. Pediatrics. 2008;121 Suppl 3:S167–71.
5. Sørensen K, Mouritsen A, Aksglaede L, Hagen CP, Mogensen SS, Juul A. Recent secular trends in pubertal timing: implications for evaluation and diagnosis of precocious puberty. Horm Res Paediatr. 2012;77(3):137–45.
6. Anderson SE, Must A. Interpreting the continued decline in the average age at menarche: results from two nationally representative surveys of U.S. girls studied 10 years apart. J Pediatr. 2005;147(6):753–60.
7. Anderson SE, Dallal GE, Must A. Relative weight and race influence average age at menarche: results from two nationally representative surveys of US girls studied 25 years apart. Pediatrics. 2003;111(4 Pt 1):844–50.
8. Marshall WA, Tanner JM. Variations in the pattern of pubertal changes in boys. Arch Dis Child. 1970;45(239):13–23.
9. Root AW. Endocrinology of puberty. I. Normal sexual maturation. J Pediatr. 1973;83(1):1–19.
10. Tanner JM, Davies PS. Clinical longitudinal standards for height and height velocity for North American children. J Pediatr. 1985;107(3):317–29.
11. Bass S, Delmas PD, Pearce G, Hendrich E, Tabensky A, Seeman E. The differing tempo of growth in bone size, mass, and density in girls is region-specific. J Clin Invest. 1999;104(6):795–804.
12. McKay HA, Bailey DA, Mirwald RL, Davison KS, Faulkner RA. Peak bone mineral accrual and age at menarche in adolescent girls: a 6-year longitudinal study. J Pediatr. 1998;133(5):682–7.

13. Whiting SJ, Vatanparast H, Baxter-Jones A, Faulkner RA, Mirwald R, Bailey DA. Factors that affect bone mineral accrual in the adolescent growth spurt. J Nutr. 2004;134(3):696S–700.
14. Abernethy L, Bleakley C. Strategies to prevent injury in adolescent sport: a systematic review. Br J Sports Med. 2007;41(10):627–38.
15. Nonfatal traumatic brain injuries related to sports and recreation activities among persons aged ≤19 years – United States, 2001–2009 [Internet]. [cited 2014 Jul 11]. Available from: http://www.cdc.gov/mmwr/preview/mmwrhtml/mm6039a1.htm.
16. Abrams GD, Renstrom PA, Safran MR. Epidemiology of musculoskeletal injury in the tennis player. Br J Sports Med. 2012;46(7):492–8.
17. Balius R, Pedret C, Estruch A, Hernández G, Ruiz-Cotorro A, Mota J. Stress fractures of the metacarpal bones in adolescent tennis players: a case series. Am J Sports Med. 2010;38(6):1215–20.
18. Lehman RC. Shoulder pain in the competitive tennis player. Clin Sports Med. 1988;7(2):309–27.
19. Alyas F, Turner M, Connell D. MRI findings in the lumbar spines of asymptomatic, adolescent, elite tennis players. Br J Sports Med. 2007;41(11):836–41. discussion 841.
20. Brenner JS. Overuse injuries, overtraining, and burnout in child and adolescent athletes. Pediatrics. 2007;119(6):1242–5.
21. Steinberg L. Cognitive and affective development in adolescence. Trends Cogn Sci. 2005;9(2):69–74.
22. Crone EA, van der Molen MW. Developmental changes in real life decision making: performance on a gambling task previously shown to depend on the ventromedial prefrontal cortex. Dev Neuropsychol. 2004;25(3):251–79.
23. Welsh MC, Pennington BF, Groisser DB. A normative-developmental study of executive function: a window on prefrontal function in children. Dev Neuropsychol. 1991;7(2):131–49.
24. Vuontela V, Steenari M-R, Carlson S, Koivisto J, Fjällberg M, Aronen ET. Audiospatial and visuospatial working memory in 6-13 year old school children. Learn Mem. 2003;10(1):74–81.
25. Mills KL, Goddings A-L, Clasen LS, Giedd JN, Blakemore S-J. The developmental mismatch in structural brain maturation during adolescence. Dev Neurosci. 2014;36(3–4):147–60.
26. Schwartz KD. Adolescent brain development: an oxymoron no longer. J Youth Minist. 2008;6(2):85–93.
27. Somerville LH, Jones RM, Casey BJ. A time of change: behavioral and neural correlates of adolescent sensitivity to appetitive and aversive environmental cues. Brain Cogn. 2010;72(1):124–33.
28. Shulman EP, Harden KP, Chein JM, Steinberg L. Sex differences in the developmental trajectories of impulse control and sensation-seeking from early adolescence to early adulthood. J Youth Adolesc. 2014;44(1):1–17.
29. Hoch AZ, Pajewski NM, Moraski L, Carrera GF, Wilson CR, Hoffmann RG, et al. Prevalence of the female athlete triad in high school athletes and sedentary students. Clin J Sport Med Off J Can Acad Sport Med. 2009;19(5):421–8.
30. Coelho GM, de O, de Farias MLF, de Mendonça LMC, de Mello DB, Lanzillotti HS, Ribeiro BG, et al. The prevalence of disordered eating and possible health consequences in adolescent female tennis players from Rio de Janeiro, Brazil. Appetite. 2013;64:39–47.
31. Mountjoy M, Sundgot-Borgen J, Burke L, Carter S, Constantini N, Lebrun C, et al. The IOC consensus statement: beyond the female athlete triad--relative energy deficiency in sport (RED-S). Br J Sports Med. 2014;48(7):491–7.
32. Goltz FR, Stenzel LM, Schneider CD. Disordered eating behaviors and body image in male athletes. Rev Bras Psiquiatr. 2013;35(3):237–42. São Paulo Braz 1999.
33. Javed A, Tebben PJ, Fischer PR, Lteif AN. Female athlete triad and its components: toward improved screening and management. Mayo Clin Proc. 2013;88(9):996–1009.
34. Sanders RA. Adolescent psychosocial, social, and cognitive development. Pediatr Rev Am Acad Pediatr. 2013;34(8):354–8. quiz 358–359.

35. Vanhalst J, Goossens L, Luyckx K, Scholte RHJ, Engels RCME. The development of loneliness from mid- to late adolescence: trajectory classes, personality traits, and psychosocial functioning. J Adolesc. 2013;36(6):1305–12.
36. Leany BD. Brain development and health implications in adolescents. In: O'Donohue WT, Benuto LT, Tolle LW, editors. Handbook of adolescent health psychology [Internet]. New York: Springer; 2013 [cited 2014 Jul 9]. p. 235–44. Available from: http://link.springer.com/chapter/10.1007/978-1-4614-6633-8_17.
37. Coatsworth JD, Conroy DE. The effects of autonomy-supportive coaching, need satisfaction, and self-perceptions on initiative and identity in youth swimmers. Dev Psychol. 2009;45(2):320–8.
38. Almagro BJ, Sáenz-López P, Moreno JA. Prediction of sport adherence through the influence of autonomy-supportive coaching among spanish adolescent athletes. J Sports Sci Med. 2010;9(1):8–14.
39. Conroy DE, Coatsworth JD. Assessing autonomy-supportive coaching strategies in youth sport. Psychol Sport Exerc. 2007;8(5):671–84.
40. Sánchez-Miguel PA, Leo FM, Sánchez-Oliva D, Amado D, García-Calvo T. The importance of Parents' behavior in their Children's enjoyment and a motivation in sports. J Hum Kinet. 2013;36:169–77.
41. Anderson JC, Funk JB, Elliott R, Smith PH. Parental support and pressure and children's extracurricular activities: relationships with amount of involvement and affective experience of participation. J Appl Dev Psychol. 2003;24(2):241–57.
42. Knight CJ, Boden CM, Holt NL. Junior tennis Players' preferences for parental behaviors. J Appl Sport Psychol. 2010;22(4):377–91.
43. Tofler IR, Knapp PK, Larden M. Achievement by proxy distortion in sports: a distorted mentoring of high-achieving youth. Historical perspectives and clinical intervention with children, adolescents, and their families. Clin Sports Med. 2005;24(4):805–28. viii.
44. Tofler IR, Knapp PK, Drell MJ. The "achievement by proxy" spectrum: recognition and clinical response to pressured and high-achieving children and adolescents. J Am Acad Child Adolesc Psychiatry. 1999;38(2):213–6.
45. Raedeke TD. Is athlete burnout more than just stress? A sport commitment perspective. J Sport Amp Exerc Psychol. 1997;19(4):396–417.
46. Breuner CC. Avoidance of burnout in the young athlete. Pediatr Ann. 2012;41(8):335–9.

Chapter 3
Mental Development in the Young Athlete

Daniel Gould and Jennifer Nalepa

The field of sport psychology focuses on the scientific study of people and their behavior in sport [1]. When applied to tennis, sport and exercise psychology knowledge helps us understand what makes tennis players tick and how to best work with them. There are two general questions sport psychologists ask: (1) what effect psychological factors have on player development and performance and (2) how participation in tennis influences the social psychological development of the participant. Hence, those interested in the psychology of tennis want to understand topics such as what motivates players; the influence that the use of psychological skills like goal setting, imagery, or confidence has on performance; the best ways for parents and coaches to help players develop; and how participation in tennis can be used to develop life skills like leadership, teamwork, discipline, and goal setting. These are skills that can be used not only on the court but off the court as well.

Because tennis tests a player as much physically as it does mentally, there is a long and rich history of applying psychological principles in tennis. Many top players have used sport psychology specialists to optimally prepare mentally, enhance their motivation, and deal with the stress of tournament play. The psychology of coaching also has a long and rich history in tennis. However, it is not just adults or elite players that need sport psychology. Applying psychology to the young athlete is critical for several reasons. First, because children differ in important ways from adults, it is critical that parents and coaches understand psychologically based development differences characterizing different age groups of children. Second, the first exposure to tennis typically occurs when one is a child and how this experience goes has much to do with long-term involvement in sport and physical activity. Finally, recent research has established that children and youth can learn important

D. Gould, PhD (✉) • J. Nalepa
Kinesiology, Institute for the Study of Youth Sports, Michigan State University,
308 W Circle Drive, Rm 201, East Lansing, MI 48824, USA
e-mail: drgould@msu.edu; nalepaje@msu.edu

© Springer International Publishing Switzerland 2016
A.C. Colvin, J.N. Gladstone (eds.), *The Young Tennis Player: Injury Prevention and Treatment,* Contemporary Pediatric and Adolescent Sports Medicine,
DOI 10.1007/978-3-319-27559-8_3

life skills like goal setting, leadership, and teamwork from participation in out-of-school extracurricular activities like sports [2, 3].

Understanding Stages of Athlete Development

Before discussing the psychological development of the young player, it is important to understand stages of athlete development, as over the last 30 years considerable research has focused on the athletic talent development process [4]. Based on this research, the United States Tennis Association (USTA) Player Development Division, in conjunction with the Sport Science Committee, has identified phases of player development based on age, experience, and level of play [5]. These stages include the:

1. *Introduction/foundation phase*, where the focus is on exposing young people, typically ages 6–12, to tennis and making the experience fun while instilling key physical and psychosocial fundamentals underlying the game. In this stage, basic movement skills like balance and jumping are emphasized as well as multisport participation. Little emphasis should be placed on rankings, winning, and competitive success. It is critical that parents and coaches are highly encouraging during this stage.
2. *Refinement/transition phase*, typically involving players ranging from 10 to 20 years of age, where the focus is on learning to train and compete. During this stage, the player shifts from wanting to play tennis to desiring to be a good player. With the help of a master coach, the player focuses on refining his or her skills.
3. *Elite world-class* performance phase, ages 15 and above, where the focus is on refining skills and pursuing excellence. Competitive excellence is emphasized and players spend many hours perfecting their skills. While a love of the game is necessary for long-term success, players realize the sport becomes a serious business.

While not all players will have the genetic gifts and/or motivation to progress through all these stages of tennis talent development, understanding these phases are important for a number of reasons. First, to have a rewarding and successful experience as a recreational player, a child needs to develop good fundamentals and a love of the game. Completing the first and perhaps the start of the second phase will equip a young person with the skills and love of the game needed to purse tennis across his or her lifespan. Given that tennis is a lifetime sport that can be pursed into one's eighties, participation has important health consequences. Second, elite players have been shown to follow this progression and most experts feel that doing so will maximize their potential. Skipping or rushing through stages is thought to thwart player development and is problematic. Finally, a professionalization of youth sports, where there is an emphasis on competition, single-sport specialization, and year-round training at very early ages, is occurring [6]. The consequences of professionalization of youth sports are that children rush or skip through the early phases of tennis development. This often results in overuse injuries [7, 8] and declines in player motivation and player burnout [9–11]. Keeping these stages in mind, then, have important implications for health professionals working with both recreational and competitive youth tennis players.

Developmentally Appropriate Tennis

Major changes have taken place in the United States on how tennis is taught to children. The USTA has reengineered how children are introduced to tennis. Historically, children have learned tennis on adult courts using adult-sized equipment with an instructor demonstrating and explaining the various strokes and then feeding balls to children one at time while the others wait in line for their turns. However, this is contrary to what motor development and sport pedagogy scholars suggest as these experts recommend that children use developmentally appropriate equipment [12] and play on courts scaled to their size and abilities. In addition, a games approach that emphasizes rally play and eliminating long lines in practice has been recommended [13]. For these reasons, the USTA developed its 10 and Under Tennis QuickStart play format [14].

The USTA's 10 and Under Tennis QuickStart play format uses smaller rackets, bigger and lighter (slower) tennis balls, smaller courts, and smaller nets. The modified equipment allows the children to more easily hit successful shots as the equipment is suited to their motor abilities and strength levels. Another method the USTA uses to make tennis more enjoyable and to improve rally performance for children is implementing a games model for teaching tennis as opposed to the traditional model. Thus, instead of the coach feeding tennis balls to each child while the others wait in line, the children play together with each other with the instructor stopping play at appropriate times and giving quick instructions. The games approach within the QuickStart format allows children opportunities to rally earlier, giving them both earlier and greater success than players who learn with the traditional format. The games approach is more fun for children since they are active for the majority of the lesson. Interestingly, several recent studies have verified the advantages of developmentally appropriate tennis over traditional adult tennis for children with modified tennis, resulting in more hitting opportunities, more hitting success, and greater happiness [12, 15].

Psychosocial Characteristics and Attributes of Developing Players

"Kids are not miniature adults" is a fundamental principle that developmental sport psychology specialists and coaching educators have and continue to convey to coaches, parents, and others working with children and youth in sport, in general, and tennis in particular [16, 17]. For this reason, it is critical that tennis parents and practitioners understand basic stages of child development and the psychological characteristics accompanying those stages. Based both on developmental psychology and sport psychology literature, a number of scholars have addressed this issue [16, 18–23] and many of the typical psychological characteristics and attributes that they use to describe children and youth of varying stages are contained in Table 3.1.

Table 3.1 Psychosocial characteristics of children and youth of varying chronological age

Age category	Psychosocial characteristics
Ages 6–8	Short attention span
	Difficulty viewing the world from the perspective of others
	Self-centered
	Developing self-esteem and self-worth but fewer subdomains seen and less differentiation
	Self-esteem and worth based on a limited number of sources
	Self-esteem and worth seen as "good" or "bad"
	Self-esteem often positive but unrealistic
	Cannot handle criticism and failure well
	At times can act out to gain attention
	Cannot differentiate effort and ability
	Limited ability to think abstractly so concrete examples needed to understand
	Frequent mood swings
	Strives to please parents and authority figures for adult approval
	Dependent on significant others for feedback
	Strict adherence to rules
Ages 9–12	Begin to recognize others' perspectives
	Starting to differentiate effort and ability and task difficulty and luck (often can do so by end of stage)
	Can better focus and make decisions but still developing in this regard
	Can better understand technical strategies
	Verbalizes thoughts and feelings
	Can talk through problems
	Wants to be with friends/trying to understand friendship with peers, especially same sex peers
	Have best friends/want to be close
	Idolizes older boys and girls
	Looks to adult authority figures for direction but starts to want independence by period end
	Starts to understand emotional processes and multiple emotions
	Active and boundless energy
	More sophisticated and realistic self-representation
	More realistic view of self
	More differentiated self-esteem
	More self-comparison regarding physical status
	Friendship predominately based on shared interests and common characteristics
	Uses peer comparisons, feedback from adults, and actual performance to judge competence
	Learns skills in parts
	Begins to see authority figures as fallible
	May defy authority
	Developing patience
	Strives to please parents but peers become more important
	Begins to be able to reflect
	Rules can be negotiated
	Behaves morally to avoid punishment

(continued)

Table 3.1 (continued)

Age category	Psychosocial characteristics
Ages 13–15	Can differentiate effort and ability and task difficulty and luck
	Better able to understand feelings of others and empathize
	Community/awareness of others and common good increases
	Concerned about feelings and being liked
	Uses multiple sources of information to define self
	Grater fluctuations in self-esteem/can have shaky self-esteem
	Works to establish self-identity
	Self-esteem vulnerable to peer pressure
	Can hurt others to feel superior
	Body dissatisfaction may appear
	Peers become very important and near peers serve as a sources of competence
	Social status dependent on group status and conformity to group norms
	Psychologically distances self from parents
	Coaches seen as more important authority figure where parents seen as less important
	Able to critically think
	More adult-like coping strategies used
	Emotional management increases
Ages 16–17	Friendship based on trust and loyalty
	Can better delay gratification
	Self-directed
	Shift toward use of internal sources of competence information
	Use personal effort to judge competence
	Can better tolerate frustration
	Challenges rules/less accepting
	Greater understanding of multiple domains of self
	More capable of expressing feelings
	Able to think abstractly so they can ponder moral dilemmas
	Wants leadership role
	Wants autonomy and to engage in decision-making
	Increase in peer and social relationships
	Peer influence begins to decline
	More likely to engage in risky behavior

It must be noted, however, that there is considerable variability within each stage as chronological age is, at best, a rough predictor for physical, psychosocial, and cognitive maturation. Practitioners must also recognize that each child develops at his or her own individual specific rate so children on the same aged-based teams can vary considerably in their characteristics and attributes. Finally, females mature faster than males, so females will enter and exit each stage slightly earlier than their male counterparts.

Remembering these psychosocial characteristics and attributes of children are important because children have different needs at each stage. In addition, they need to be parented or coached differently at the differing stages of development.

Motivation for Tennis Involvement and Withdrawal

Understanding why children participate in sport, as well as their reasons for withdrawal, has been a topic of considerable interest in sport and exercise psychology. While the bulk of the research focuses on youth sports in general, some studies have focused on the young tennis player's motives for participation [24, 25] and withdrawal [26]. In general, the tennis-specific studies parallel the research on other sports.

Among the motives cited for tennis involvement, fun, physical fitness, improving skills, and making and being with friends are the motives most often cited by children and youth [25, 27]. The general youth sport research also reveals that youth have multiple motives for participation. Relative to gender, males and females are more similar than different, although males more often cited competitive motives like competition, status, and earning awards, while females indicated more affiliation-related motives [1, 27]. Older tennis playing children (ages 12 and above) more often cited being popular, being with friends, satisfying parents, and using equipment as major motives more than younger participants and most importantly, young players cited perceiving their roles positively and good coach relations as more important motives for play [27].

Researchers have also examined motives for sport withdrawal. Specifically looking at tennis and paralleling research with young athletes in other youth sports, "having other things to do" is the most often-cited reasoning for discontinuing involvement [28]. This is not surprising as many young athletes sample different youth sports before settling in on those sports they are most interested in or unfortunately drop out of sport altogether. In addition, children often need to select between multiple desirable activities like going to scouts or tennis because they meet at the same time. "Other things to do" also sometimes masks other motives such as low perceived competence or not being as good as one wants to be. Lastly, other motives often cited for youth tennis withdrawal include dislike of the coach, perceived failure and a lack of a team atmosphere/spirit, no team work, and not as good as wanted to be [28]. These later motives are particularly important because parents and coaches can greatly influence them through the sport environments they create.

It has been suggested that while the above findings provide the descriptive reasons children give for sport participation and withdrawal, these are more surface-related motives. Underlying these surface motives are deeper motives [1]. These include perceived competence, achievement goals and goal orientations, and self-determined motivation.

One of the most consistent findings in the youth sports literature focuses on perceived competence or how children and youth view themselves physically, socially, and cognitively [17]. Simply put, young athletes who perceive themselves to be physically competent are much more likely to participate in sport than children who do not. In addition, children are more likely to discontinue sport involvement if they perceive they lack physical competence. These findings suggest, then, that one way to enhance and maintain youth tennis participation is to find ways to help children feel physically competent as enhanced skills are correlated to improved competence [24]. Interestingly, helping more children rally sooner and have more early success is a key rationale behind the initiation of the 10 and Under Tennis QuickStart format. A number of effective coaching strategies have also been identified for enhancing perceived competence in young athletes like helping match tasks to participant capabilities and helping players define success on self-improvement [24].

Achievement goal orientations focus on how people view success in achievement-related activities, like tennis [29]. An ego orientation focuses on defining success by comparing oneself to others via social comparison, for example, by winning a match or establishing a particular ranking. With a task orientation, one focuses on defining success by making comparisons to one's own or self-referenced standards like improving on their previous performances or mastering certain shots and skills. A wealth of research reveals that young athletes, including tennis players, who adopt a task versus ego orientation, sustain motivation, persist longer at activities, select more challenging tasks, exhibit less anxiety, and experience greater satisfaction from play [29, 30].

Related to the idea of achievement goal orientations is research on motivational climates or what training and competitive environments are created by significant others and coaches [29, 31]. A task or mastery-oriented climate emphasizes self-improvement, cooperation, and positive group relations, whereas an ego or outcome-focused climate emphasizes results and outcomes, a focus on competition between players, rivalry, and recognizing more talented individuals. The research reveals that young players who participate in task-oriented motivational climates demonstrate higher perceived competence, better work ethics, greater persistence, enjoyment, and effort [27].

Finally, one of the most popular and applied motivation theories in contemporary psychology is self-determination theory [32], and this theory has been tested and applied to the sport context [33, 34]. According to this view, individuals can be intrinsically or extrinsically motivated with intrinsic motivation focusing on self-determined reasons for participation like self-satisfaction or individual improvement and extrinsic motivation focusing on external reasons for participation like receiving tangible rewards for participation or participating to please others. While most children, and people in general, are not purely intrinsically or extrinsically motivated, playing for intrinsic versus extrinsic reasons results in a number of motivational benefits. For this reason, most sport psychologists feel the use of external rewards should not be overused with young players as they can easily be seen as controlling one's behavior which results in a decline of intrinsic motivation when the rewards are not present. Instead, intrinsic reasons for participation should be emphasized.

Another component of self-determination theory is the identification of three basic needs that drive human behavior [35]. These include: the need to feel competent, the need for relatedness, and the need to have personal autonomy. Research suggests that the more a young player can feel he or she is competent, has his or her relatedness needs met (enjoys his or her training group), and is given choices relative to his or her tennis (e.g., be given a choice about what they practice or what tournaments he or she might attend), the more he or she will be motivated [34].

Player Stress and Burnout

Are young athletes placed under too much stress? Is early sports specialization causing talented young tennis players to burnout of the sport? How can we prepare young tennis players to deal with the physical and psychological demands of competitive tennis? These are just some of the questions that those in sports medicine, coaching, and related professions are asked on a frequent basis. While sport psychological research has not been able to definitively answer these questions as they relate to youth tennis involvement, considerable evidence has been amassed in pediatric sport science research that helps provide answers. Some of this evidence will now be reviewed.

There are a number of ways stress can be viewed. Sport psychology researchers have defined stress as a process that occurs when an individual, in our case a developing player, perceives that some physical or psychological demands exceeds his or her response capabilities under conditions where meeting that demand has important consequences [1]. When stress is perceived, it results in a psychophysiological reaction (e.g., increased muscle tension, racing heart, state anxiety, or right-now feelings of tension and worry) that influences both performance and affect. Physical and psychological demands (stressors) include such things as having to train for two hours every day, traveling to tournaments every weekend, trying to meet one's parents' expectations for success, and/or dealing with a disappointing tournament loss. However, stressors are not the only causes of anxiety and stress. An individual's personality characteristics shape the way he or she perceives potential demanding or stressful situations. For example, a low self-esteem and high trait anxious (a predisposition to perceive evaluative environments as threatening) young player will perceive the same environment (e.g., playing in a big tournament, closing out a close match) as more stressful and respond with more state anxiety than a player with high self-esteem and low trait anxiety). Hence, two young players can have vastly different reactions to the same potentially threatening or stressful situation.

With the above being said, sport psychology research has examined sources of stress in young athletes. While there are literally hundreds of specific stressors, two general ones have been identified: the importance placed on performance and the uncertainty regarding outcomes [36]. Specifically, the greater the importance a young athlete perceives is placed on his or her performance or tennis play, the more anxiety is experienced. Similarly, the more uncertainty one has about his or her capabilities to cope with the demands placed on him or her, the more stress is experienced. This suggests that parents and coaches need to be very careful about placing too much importance on the outcomes of tennis matches (e.g., "you need to win this one," "everyone is counting on you") and that the confidence of and coping capabilities of young players needs to be enhanced. Interestingly, one recent study showed that the more money parents paid for their child to participate in sport, the more anxiety a child experienced, suggesting that parents subtly or not so subtly conveyed that performing well was so important because participation costs so much [37].

A frequently asked question in youth sports is whether participation creates too much stress for the young participants. The good news is that research reveals that most young athletes are not placed under too much stress. However, certain children in certain situations do experience high levels of stress. The psychological characteristics of players who are at risk of being incapable of handling stress include children who are characterized by high trait anxiety, have low self-esteem, are inexperienced, adopt an outcome goal orientation, have low perceived competence, and perceive parental pressure to participate or perform [1]. Efforts must, therefore, be made to understand each player as an individual and treat them differently (e.g., de-emphasize the importance of performance and make special efforts to build confidence for players who are at risk for ill effects of stress).

Closely associated with the topic of stress in young athletes is burnout. Burnout occurs when a player psychologically and physically withdraws, loses motivation, and/or lessens involvement in an activity that was previously viewed as enjoyable as a result of chronic stress [38]. Players who experience burnout in sport are characterized by reduced sense of accomplishment, emotional and physical exhaustion, and sport devaluation [39]. The good news is that rates of burnout in young players are estimated to be very low. However, it certainly occurs and has been documented in tennis. In addition, as is the case with stress and anxiety, burnout occurs as a result of both external demands placed on a player and his or her personality and resources available for coping with the demands placed on him or her. Research conducted with junior tennis players who burned out of tennis, for example, showed that burnout could be driven by external demands (e.g., physical overtraining combined with a lack of recovery), by maladaptive perfectionistic personality (players who constantly set high standards while simultaneously being predisposed to constantly worry about mistakes), and/or by parent and coach pressure [10, 11]. In this research, players who burned out also provided advice for preventing burnout. For parents of players, they suggested that parents provide support, demonstrate empathy, reduce the importance they place on competitive outcomes, and recognize that there is an optimal amount of parental push needed. Coaches were advised to foster two-way communication with their player, solicit and use player input, work to understand player feelings, and cultivate personal relations and involvement with players. Finally, it was recommended that players themselves keep it fun, play for their own reasons, balance tennis with other pursuits, and take time off to relax.

Best Coaching Practices

Coaches are considered to be one of the most significant individuals influencing young athletes. For this reason, researchers have examined effective coaching practices specifically as they relate to young developing athletes. This research reveals that children have different coaching needs than adults and that certain coaching practices and behaviors are related to optimal development in young athletes [40].

The seminal research in this area was conducted by Smith, Smoll, and their colleagues who, in series of field and intervention studies, found specific links between coaching behaviors like reinforcement, punishment, and technical instruction and youth outcomes like player self-esteem, anxiety, and motivation for participation [40]. For example, in a study of 52 youth baseball coaches and over 500 of their players, it was found that positive reinforcement and encouraging players after mistakes were associated with postseason self-esteem measures, liking of teammates, and liking of baseball. It was also found that coaches who gave technical instruction were viewed more positively by their players than coaches who used general communication and encouragement [41]. In a follow-up intervention study, it was found that coaches trained to be more encouraging and less punitive had players rate them as better teachers. The players who played for these coaches also indicated that they both liked their coaches and teammates more and showed greater positive changes in self-esteem. Subsequent studies further verified and built upon these initial findings showing that coaches who were taught a positive and encouraging approach to coaching had lower player dropout rates across the season [42] and that a positive mastery-oriented approach to coaching was related to decreases in player anxiety over the course of a playing season [43]. Finally, in a recent review of all the research in this area, Langan, Blake, and Longsdale concluded that these programs enhance the interpersonal effectiveness of coaches [44]. Changes in coaching behaviors are also linked to personal and social outcomes in the coaches' young athletes, and there is no evidence that these interventions have any harmful effects.

The coaching effectiveness research leads to a number of practical guidelines for coaching young athletes [1]. These include avoiding punitive, controlling, and hostile coaching behaviors while emphasizing positive, encouraging, and autonomy-supportive behaviors. When giving encouraging remarks, make sure they are given sincerely and convey specific information. Coaches should also reward effort as much as outcomes and create environments where young athletes do not fear making mistakes. Lastly, provide plenty of instruction and increase the chances of player success by modifying skills and activities so they are developmentally appropriate.

Best Parenting Practices

A topic of considerable practical interest in youth tennis is the role of parents in initiating and supporting their child's play. Much of the reason for this concern is because of highly visible examples of inappropriate parental behavior resulting with tennis parents being barred from competitions or being brought up on criminal charges for attacking opponents. This mirrors increased concerns with parents across all youth sports.

Luckily, over the last several decades, considerable research has been conducted on the role parents play in youth sports with much of the research being conducted on tennis parents. In a survey study conducted with a national sample of junior tennis coaches, Gould, Lauer, Rolo, Jannes, and Pennisi found that six out of ten parents were seen as having positive influence on their child's tennis development [45]. Thus, the majority of tennis parents do not interfere with their child's development. In fact, sport-parenting research supports the idea that parents play a crucial role in their child's youth sport experience in three important ways. These include: (1) as providers of the sport experience by doing such things as transporting children to and from games and practices and paying for lessons; (2) as role models who vicariously provide information about sport involvement, it's importance, and how to interact with those in sport; and (3) as interpreters of their sport experience by influencing such factors as their children's perceptions of competence and stress levels through the expectations they hold and importance they place on success [46]. Thus, parent involvement is essential to a productive youth sports experience.

Not all parents' behaviors have positive influences, however. Three out of every ten parents are viewed by coaches as interfering with their child's development by exhibiting such attitudes and behaviors as overemphasizing winning, holding unrealistic expectations, coaching the child when not a coach, criticizing the child, pampering the child too much, and pushing the child to play [47].

While a comprehensive review of all the youth sports parenting research is beyond the scope of this review, the USTA commissioned the Institute for the Study of Youth Sports at Michigan State University to review all the sport-parenting research [48]. The tennis-specific research conclusions of that review follow.

1. Parents play a critical role in their child's tennis experience. They provide a wide variety of support ranging from financial and logistical support to emotional–social support [49]. In fact, they make a number of sacrifices so their children can develop in the sport [45, 47].
2. Tennis parents create psychological climates, hold various attitudes and values, form expectations, and emit certain behaviors and actions that have major influences on their child's psychological development. Specifically, Harwood and Swain showed that parents have a major influence on the development and activation of their child's achievement goals [50]. Fathers often created ego climates and pressured their children. Moreover, based on their findings, these investigators suggested that parents must pay particular attention to preventing their child from playing in an ego-oriented climate, especially if they are under 12 years of age since children under this age will become immersed in social comparison since developmentally they have trouble setting self-referenced standards on their own. Researchers have also shown that parental pressure is associated with increased state anxiety in young athletes [51], as well as the development of important personality dispositions such as perfectionism [52]. Conversely, low parental pressure is associated with increased player satisfaction [51].
3. The majority of tennis parents have been found to possess attitudes and values and do things that facilitate their child's overall and tennis talent development in a positive manner. However, research also shows that a significant minority of tennis parents hold attitudes or emit actions that inhibit their child's development. For example, De Francesco and Johnson found that 29 % of players felt

their parents behaved inappropriately by doing such things as walking away from the court, screaming or yelling at them, or even hitting them [53]. These findings are disturbing and need to be addressed.

4. A number of tennis parental actions and behaviors have been associated with positive and negative player development. Positive behaviors that have been identified include providing a wide variety of support ranging from transportation and financial to social and emotional, holding emotionally intelligent discussions with their child, focusing on the child's psychological and social development, as well as tennis development, maintaining a positive perspective by focusing on performance versus outcome goals, adopting a long-term focus on player development, staying calm and controlling emotions, and reducing pressure on their player [45, 47, 54]. Behaviors associated with negative player development included adopting a winning-only focus, attempting to control their child's involvement, being overinvolved and pushing their child, engaging in critical and negative communication, verbal and physical abuse, overemphasizing winning and player development, placing tennis above total child development, and using controlling behaviors [45, 47, 54]. Knight, Holden, and Bolt also found that players preferred that their parents comment on their effort and attitude, provide practical advice, respect tennis etiquette, and match on verbal behaviors with supportive comments [55]. They also preferred that their parents not provide technical and tactical advice.

5. Parental involvement and the specific behaviors and actions needed are dependent on the stage of athletic development. Tennis parents are most involved in the early years of play (under the age of 12 years) with their involvement lessening in the teenage years. Moreover, the types and quality of involvement change over time with most parents exhibiting supportive behaviors in the early years of involvement and more pressure-related, pushy, and controlling behaviors in the middle years of involvement [54].

6. Parental pressure and player perceptions of pressure from their parents have been shown to have negative effects on player affective states and involvement [51]. Parental pressure has also been identified as one of a number of causes of player burnout [9–11]. Research by Bois, Lalanne, and Dulforge has also shown that female players have been found to be especially vulnerable to stress [51]. Finally, these investigators have also found that directive and controlling parental behaviors have been found to be most often linked to heightened player anxiety.

7. The tennis parenting experience has also been found to be stressful. Chief sources of parental stress included competition, coaches, finances, siblings, time organization related, and developmental [56]. Moreover, parents were found to experience a diverse array of stressors before, during, and post match. In a second study, three categories of parental stressors were identified. These included: organizational stressors related to time demands, finance, training, and coaching; competitive stressors tied to performance issues and morality issues associated with match play; and developmental stressors including issues associated with the child's education, tennis transitions, and future [56]. It has also been found

that parents in the initial stage of athlete development experienced the fewest stressors. Organizational stressors were most prevalent in the specializing and investment stages of player development. Based on these findings, it was suggested that parents need assistance in ways to cope with the stressors associated with tennis parenting.

8. Tennis talent development is associated with certain parenting practices and actions. Lauer and his associates found that professional tennis players, whose transitions through stages of athletic talent development were characterized as smooth, difficult, or tumultuous, reported experiencing differing types of sport parenting [57]. Players who reported smooth transitions had parents who were predominately supportive, while difficult and tumultuous transition players reported more conflicts with parents and negative parent–child interactions. Finally, the notion of optimal parent push has been identified in several tennis parenting studies conducted by Gould, Lauer, and their colleagues [47, 54, 57]. While more research is needed before we can definitively understand optimal parent push, the research conducted to date suggests that it involves holding the player accountable and stressing core values like hard work, discipline, and sportsmanship while placing little importance on rankings and winning. Non-optimal push involves placing winning and rankings above player development and engaging in controlling, negative, and critical parental behaviors. In addition, non-optimal push might be characterized by too little involvement in the child's tennis where inadequate support is provided.

Finally, the USTA Player Development Division has developed several tennis parent education power point sessions that coaches and sports medicine professionals can download and use to educate tennis parents. One is designed for parents whose children are just beginning the game [58] and the second for parents of players involved in competitive junior tennis [59]. Both these guides are available at no cost.

Psychological Skills Development in Children

Psychological skills training focuses on the systematic teaching and learning of mental skills that can be used to help athletes better meet their sport goals [1]. The fostering of psychological skills in developing players is important for a number of reasons. First, as a child progresses through the stages of athletic talent development, they will need to cope with more pressure and demands associated with competitive play. It is also important to note that confidence issues and anxiety effects can occur with children at any level of play. Second, high life stress has been shown to be one of the most consistent psychological predictors of athletic injuries for young athletes with low coping skills and social support being most particularly vulnerable to the life stress injury relationship [60]. So teaching young athletes coping skills along with insuring adequate social support may help prevent some injuries. Third, psychology of injury research shows that athletes can use a number of psychological skills like relaxation strategies, imagery, goal setting, and self-talk to facilitate recovery [61, 62]. Young athletes who learn these skills as part of their tennis training will be better equipped to transfer them for use if they become injured. Finally, recent research shows that psychological skills and attributes learned in sport can be transferred beyond sport to facilitate development and performance in other life pursuits [63]. However, this life skills development best occurs when those skills are intentionally fostered in the sport experience. In other words, they are more taught than caught!

We are not suggesting that every young tennis player needs to seek out and see a sport psychology specialist, although some may need to do so (e.g., high trait anxious player with low coping skills suffering from the debilitating effects of stress). However, coaches can teach mental skills as part of the tennis experience, and resources exist to help them do so [64]. Lauer and his colleagues, for instance, have outlined key steps for coaching mental skills which include: (1) identifying mental skills needs of the athlete, (2) determining mental skills training goals and setting a mental skills training schedule, (3) planning how to integrate mental skills training into practices, (4) implementing the training prior to the season or away from competition, and (5) evaluating athlete mental skills progress and adapting the program based on this feedback [64]. Recent research has also supported the efficacy of mental skills training for young athletes [65, 66].

When fostering mental skills in young players, developmental differences characterizing children of different ages should be kept in mind. For example, an 8-year-old player who is characterized by concrete thinking cannot understand anxiety as an adult might. However, he or she can understand that making his or her body feel like warm-cooked spaghetti might help deal with anxiety, or he or she can understand slow rhythmic berating by practicing bubble blowing [21, 67]. Visek, Harris, and Blom also suggest that clear and simple language be used with children and sessions reduced from an hour to 20–30 min and be held more frequently [21]. Repetition may be needed to facilitate memory while creating smaller workgroups to avoid peer pressure.

Summary

Tennis is a lifetime sport that has many potential physical, psychological, and social benefits for children and youth. However, these benefits will only occur if children and youth have positive and fulfilling initial experiences in the sport. Knowledge from the psychology of sport and exercise has much to offer coaches and parents who want to provide for such optimal experiences. However, coaches and parents remain largely uneducated about these topics. Health-care providers, therefore, can play an important role in educating parents in regard to the best ways to foster optimal mental development of the young player and in so doing enhance overall psychological and physical health.

References

1. Weinberg R, Gould D. Foundations of sport and exercise psychology. 6th ed. Champaign: Human Kinetics; 2015.
2. Gould D, Carson S. Young athlete's perceptions of the relationship between coaching behaviors and development experiences. Int J Coaching Sci. 2011;5(2):3–29.
3. Larson R, Hansen D, Moneta G. Differing profiles of developmental experiences across types of organized youth activities. Dev Psychol. 2006;42(5):849–63.
4. Gould D, Cowburn I. The role of psychological factors in the development of Olympic athletes. In: Zinchencko Y, Hanin J, editors. Sport psychology: on the Way to the Olympic games. 1st ed. Moscow: Moscow State University; 2013.
5. Gould D, Lubbers P. The progressive development of the high performance player. High Perform Coach. 2004;6(1):5–8.
6. Gould D. The professionalization of youth sports: it's time to act! Clin J Sports Med. 2009;19:81–2.
7. Brenner J. Overuse injuries, overtraining, and burnout in child and adolescent athletes. Pediatrics. 2007;119(6):1242–5.
8. Hutchinson M, Laprade R, Burnett Q, Moss R, Terpstra J. Injury surveillance at the USTA Boys' Tennis Championships: a 6-yr study. Med Sci Sports Exerc. 1995;27(6):826–31.
9. Gould D, Udry E, Tuffey S, Loehr J. Burnout in competitive junior tennis players, I: a quantitative psychological assessment. Sport Psychol. 1996;10:322–40.
10. Gould D, Tuffey S, Udry E, Loehr J. Burnout in competitive junior tennis players, II: qualitative analysis. Sport Psychol. 1996;10:341–66.
11. Gould D, Tuffey S, Udry E, Loehr J. Burnout in competitive junior tennis players, III: individual differences in the burnout experience. Sport Psychol. 1997;11:257–76.
12. Buszard T, Farrow D, Reid M, Masters R. Modifying equipment in early skill development: a tennis perspective. Res Q Exerc Sport. 2014;85(2):218–25.
13. Turner A, Martinek T. An investigation into teaching games for understanding: effects on skill, knowledge, and game play. Res Q Exerc Sport. 1999;70(3):286–96.
14. Anderson K, Davis A, Cleland S, Jamision J, Avischious G, Murren M. Quickstart tennis: an exciting new play format for kids 10 and under. Whiteplans: USTA; 2009.
15. Farrow D, Reid M. The effect of equipment scaling on the skill acquisition of beginning tennis players. J Sport Sci. 2010;28(7):723–32.
16. Haneline B. Positioning youth tennis for success. White Plains: United States Tennis Association; 2013.
17. Weiss M, Ferrer-Caja E. Motivational orientations and sport behavior. In: Horn T, editor. Advances in sport psychology. 1st ed. Champaign: Human Kinetics; 2002. p. 101–84.
18. Developmental milestones chart. 1st ed. The Institute for Human Services for The Ohio Child Welfare Training Program; 2008.
19. Daniels A, Perkins D, Stern M. Putting youth back into sports [Brookings, South Dakota]. South Dakota State University, College of Agricultural & Biological Sciences, Cooperative Extension Service; 2003.
20. Thompson R, Winer A, Goodwin R. The individual child: temperament, emotion, self, and personality. In: Lamb M, Bornstein M, editors. Social and personality development. 1st ed. New York: Psychology Press; 2011. p. 217–58.
21. Visek A, Harris B, Blom L. Mental training with youth sport teams: developmental considerations and best-practice recommendations. J Sport Psychol Act. 2013;4(1):45–55.
22. Vernon A. Working with children, adolescents and their parents: practical application of developmental theory. In: Vernon A, editor. Counseling children and adolescents. 1st ed. Denver: Love Publishing; 2004. p. 1–34.
23. Weiss M. Developmental sport and exercise psychology: a lifespan approach. Morgantown: Fitness Information Technology; 2004.

24. Ebbeck V. Self-perception and motivational characteristics of tennis participants: the influence of age and skill. J Appl Sport Psychol. 1994;6(1):71–86.
25. Kolt G, Capaldi R. Why do children participate in tennis? ACHPER Healthy Lifestyles J. 2001;48(2):9–13.
26. Alvarez E, Marquez S. Dropout reasons in young Spanish athletes: relationship to gender, type of sport and level of competition. J Sport Behav. 2006;29(3):255–269.
27. Crespo M, Reid M. Motivation in tennis. Br J Sports Med. 2007;21:6–21.
28. Molinero O, Salguero A, Álvarez E, Márquez S. Reasons for dropout in youth soccer: a comparison with other team sports. Eur J Hum Mov. 2010;22:21–30.
29. Duda J. Motivation in sport: the relevance of competence and achievement goals. In: Elliot A, Dweck C, editors. Handbook of competence and motivation. 1st ed. New York: Guilford Press; 2005. p. 318–35.
30. Van de Pol P, Kavussanu M. Achievement goals and motivational responses in tennis: does the context matter? Psychol Sport Exercise. 2011;12(2):176–83.
31. Ntoumanis N, Biddle S. A review of psychological climate in physical activity settings with specific reference to motivation. J Sport Sci. 1999;17:643–65.
32. Deci E, Ryan R. Intrinsic motivation and self-determination in human behavior. New York: Plenum; 1985.
33. Cervelló E, Santos Rosa F, Calvo T, Jiménez R, Iglesias D. Young tennis players' competitive task involvement and performance: the role of goal orientations, contextual motivational climate, and coach-initiated motivational climate. J Appl Sport Psychol. 2007;19(3):304–21.
34. Vallerand R, Losier G. An integrative analysis of intrinsic and extrinsic motivation in sport. J Appl Sport Psychol. 1999;11(1):142–69.
35. Ryan R, Deci E. Self-determination theory and the facilitation of intrinsic motivation, social development, and well-being. Am Psychol. 2000;55(1):68–78.
36. Martens R. Joy and sadness in children's sports. Champaign: Human Kinetics Publishers; 1978.
37. Dorsch T, Lowe K, Dotterer A. NCAA innovations grant. Nat Collegiate Athletic Assoc. 2014;2014:1–47.
38. Gould D, Whitley M. Sources and consequences of athletic burnout among college athletes. J Intercollegiate Athlet. 2009;2:16–30.
39. Raedeke T, Smith A. Development and preliminary validation of an athlete burnout measure. J Sport Exercise Psychol. 2001;23:281–306.
40. Smoll FL, Smith RE. Mastery approach to coaching: a leadership guide for youth sports. Seattle: Y-E-Sports; 2009.
41. Smith R, Smoll F, Curtis S. Coach effectiveness training: a cognitive-behavioral approach to enhancing relationship skills in youth sport coaches. J Sport Psychol. 1979;1:59–75.
42. Barnett N, Smoll F, Smith R. Effects of enhancing coach-athlete relationships on youth sport attrition. Sport Psychol. 1992;6:111–27.
43. Smith R, Smoll F, Cumming S. Effects of a motivational climate intervention for coaches on young athlete' sport performance anxiety. J Sport Exercise Psychol. 2007;29:39–59.
44. Langan E, Blake C, Lonsdale C. Systematic review of the effectiveness of interpersonal coach education interventions on athlete outcomes. Psychol Sport Exercise. 2013;14(1):37–49.
45. Gould D, Lauer L, Rolo C, Jannes C, Pennisi N. Understanding the role parents play in tennis success: a national survey of junior tennis coaches. Br J Sports Med. 2006;40:632–6.
46. Fredricks J, Eccles J. Parental influences on youth involvement in sports. In: Weiss M, editor. Developmental sport and exercise psychology: a lifespan perspective. 1st ed. Morgantown: Information Technology; 2015.
47. Gould D, Lauer L, Rolo C, Jannes C, Pennisi N. The role of parents in tennis success: focus group interviews with junior coaches. Sport Psychol. 2008;22(1):18–27.
48. Gould D, Cowburn I, Pierce S. Sport parenting research: current status, future directions, and practical implications. US Tennis Association White Paper Report. Boca Raton, Florida: US Tennis Association; 2012.

49. Wolfenden L, Holt N. Talent development in elite junior tennis: perceptions of players, parents, and coaches. J Appl Sport Psychol. 2005;17(2):108–26.
50. Harwood C, Swain A. The development and activation of achievement goals in tennis: I. Understanding the underlying factors. Sport Psychol. 2001;15(3):319–41.
51. Bois J, Lalanne J, Delforge C. The influence of parenting practices and parental presence on children's and adolescents' pre-competitive anxiety. J Sports Sci. 2009;27(10):995–1005.
52. Appleton P, Hall H, Hill A. Family patterns of perfectionism: an examination of elite junior athletes and their parents. Psychol Sport Exercise. 2010;11(5):363–71.
53. Defrancesco C, Johnson P. Athlete and parent perceptions in junior tennis. J Sport Behav. 1997;20(1):29–36.
54. Lauer L, Gould D, Roman N, Pierce M. Parental behaviors that affect junior tennis player development. Psychol Sport Exercise. 2010;11(6):487–96.
55. Knight C, Boden C, Holt N. Junior tennis players' preferences for parental behaviors. J Appl Sport Psychol. 2010;22(4):377–91.
56. Harwood C, Knight C. Understanding parental stressors: an investigation of British tennis-parents. J Sports Sci. 2009;27(4):339–51.
57. Lauer L, Gould D, Roman N, Pierce M. How parents influence junior tennis players' development: qualitative narratives. J Clini Sport Psychol. 2010;4(1):69–92.
58. USTA Parents' Guide 1 [Internet]. 1st ed. United States Tennis Association; 2015. [Cited 15 May 2015]. Available from: http://s3.amazonaws.com/ustaassets/assets/1/usta_import/usta/dps/doc_437_1.pdf.
59. USTA Parent's Guide II [Internet]. 1st ed. United States Tennis Association; 2015. [Cited 15 May 2015]. Available from: http://s3.amazonaws.com/ustaassets/assets/1/usta_import/usta/dps/doc_437_2.pdf.
60. Smith R, Smoll F, Ptacek J. Conjunctive moderator variables in vulnerability and resiliency research: life stress, social support and coping skills, and adolescent sport injuries. J Pers Soc Psychol. 1990;58(2):360–70.
61. Cupal D, Brewer B. Effects of relaxation and guided imagery on knee strength, reinjury anxiety, and pain following anterior cruciate ligament reconstruction. Rehabil Psychol. 2001;46(1):28–43.
62. Evans L, Hardy L, Fleming S. Intervention strategies with injured athletes: an action research study. Sport Psychol. 2000;14(2):188–206.
63. Camiré M, Trudel P, Forneris T. Coaching and transferring life skills: philosophies and strategies used by model high school coaches. Sport Psychol. 2012;26(2):243.
64. Lauer L, Gould D, Lubbers P, Kovacs M. USTA mental skills and drills handbook. Monterey: Coaches Choice; 2010.
65. Gucciardi D, Gordon S, Dimmock J. Evaluation of a mental toughness training program for youth-aged Australian footballers: I. A quantitative analysis. J Appli Sport Psychol. 2009;21(3):307–23.
66. Sheard M, Golby J. Effect of a psychological skills training program on swimming performance and positive psychological development. Int J Sport Exercise Psychol. 2006;4(2):149–69.
67. Orlick T. Feeling great: teaching children to excel at living. Carp: Creative Bound; 2004.

Chapter 4
Strength and Conditioning for the Young Tennis Player

Mark S. Kovacs

Introduction

Strength and conditioning training for the young tennis player requires the progressive, age- and stage-appropriate training in the major physical aspects of athletic performance. These areas include balance, coordination, agility, running, jumping, throwing, strength, power, endurance, and flexibility. To structure an effective strength and conditioning program for tennis, the technical and physical skills needed to succeed on the tennis court are developed at different levels before, during, and after puberty all the way into early adulthood. It is important to effectively understand the demands of tennis to correctly structure an effective strength and conditioning program for the young tennis player. Before being able to effectively structure a strength and conditioning program for tennis, an understanding of the demands and injuries should be reviewed.

Junior Tennis Player Injuries

Junior tennis injuries are starting to get more media attention as youth sport injuries have increased over the past decade, and it is becoming more common to see surgeries performed on young athletes for overuse injuries. Much of this media attention stems from other sports like baseball and football, but tennis is also one sport where overuse injuries are an area that every coach, parent, Tennis Performance Trainer

M.S. Kovacs, PhD, FACSM, CTPS, MTPS, CSCS*D
Life Sport Science Institute and Department of Sport Health Science, Life University,
Marietta, GA, USA
e-mail: kovacsma@hotmail.com

© Springer International Publishing Switzerland 2016
A.C. Colvin, J.N. Gladstone (eds.), *The Young Tennis Player: Injury Prevention and Treatment*, Contemporary Pediatric and Adolescent Sports Medicine,
DOI 10.1007/978-3-319-27559-8_4

(TPT), and Certified Tennis Performance Specialist (CTPS) should have a strong education. Many of these injuries, and even surgeries, used to be only performed on college and adult athletes. Fortunately for tennis, the average young tennis player experiences relatively few severe injuries, and it is considerably lower than many other sports [1]. However, overuse is a concern in competitive young tennis athletes. Although injury rates and types of injuries are not as well researched as in some other sports (i.e., baseball, soccer, etc.), some interesting data exists that can help us better understand young tennis athletes and the typical issues they see. Over a multiyear period in a major junior national tennis tournament, 21 % of participants sustained an injury [2]. Over the last few decades, research has been inconsistent about where the majority of tennis injuries occur. Earlier research showed that a large percentage of injuries occurred in the lower body [3]. However, other research has showed that upper body and core injuries are becoming more common [4]. This is likely due to the change in technique (more open stance movements and greater reliance of upper body in stroke production, the slower surfaces) and new technologies in the racket and strings.

One unique study involved a series of questions on training, technique, competition, and other factors that were provided to all participants at the largest junior team tennis event in the USA [5]. It was collected at 12 different locations and 861 junior tennis players completed the survey:

- 97 % of individuals who completed the study
- Gender breakdown:

    Males – 43 % (356)
    Females – 57 % ($N=476$)

- Age: 10–17

As the goal of the study was to evaluate injury patterns and trends, a clear definition of injury was important: "an event that forces a player to miss 3 or more consecutive days of tennis play, either practice or competition, or that requires medical attention from a trainer, therapist, or doctor."

Major findings from this study
For both the 12 and under and 14 and under age groups, the shoulder was the most often injured area. However for the 16 and under age group, the back was the most commonly injured area
Only 51 and 54 % (male and female) of respondents use free weights and only 38 and 39 % use machines
Only 43 and 58 % (male and female) use medicine ball during training
90 and 97 % (male and female) use a double-handed backhand
20 and 22 % (male and female) use an abbreviated/short service motion
83 % of all players predominantly train and play on a hard court surface
81 % of all injuries in junior tennis players were tennis related
51 % of all athletes that reported an injury visited a physician or physical therapist

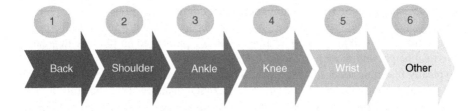

Basic Terminology

Having a good understanding of the needs of the sport helps when designing effective tennis-specific strength and conditioning programs for the young athlete. A *jump* involves a takeoff from one or both feet and a landing on both feet simultaneously [6]. A *leap* (sometimes called a bound) occurs from taking off on one foot and landing on the other [6]. A *hop* is when the takeoff and landing occur on the same single foot [6]. Other common athletic skills that need to be prioritized (especially before puberty) are the gallop, shuffle, and skip. *Galloping* and *shuffling* are a combination of a step and leap, whereas *skipping* requires combining a step with a hop [6]. Upper body actions are not as easy to distinguish as lower body actions. However, throwing and tossing are distinct. *Throwing* actions will be considered when an overhand movement is used to propel an object, while a *toss* occurs when an underhand action is employed [6]. In tennis throwing is a vital skill to help with coordination needed to perform the tennis serve and tennis overhead. Tossing is important for the development of dexterity, coordination, and the ability to use and control the upper limbs. Moving from the ground to the air and back down to the ground can be accomplished by three major movement patterns – jumping, leaping, and hopping. All individuals who are active develop these movements in activities of daily living, but very few in the current environment develop these skills to an optimum level. Some will perfect them later in life due to coaching from more knowledgeable instructors. For an in-depth explanation of jumping, leaping, and hopping mechanics, please see the following references [7, 8].

Vertical jumping can begin as early as 2 years of age [8]. Many steps are involved in the developmental transition from inefficient jumping actions to proficient movement skills. In younger or inexperienced jumpers, there is only a small preparatory countermovement action. Full extension of the hips, knees, and ankles does not fully occur at the youngest ages. Often the legs are tucked (knee flexion) under during the flight phase, so the center of mass is not elevated [6]. Another characteristic is that there is difficulty jumping and landing on both feet. A small step can usually be observed when a one-footed takeoff and landing occurs. Arm action is also asymmetrical and is not necessarily coordinated with the body or legs. Mature jumping patterns differ dramatically, and changes will occur quickly. For example, there is an appropriate preparatory countermovement action of the legs that is followed by a more forceful extension of the hips, knees, and ankles [8].

Horizontal leaping (or bounding) is another common jumping skill that is similar to running in that there is an air phase when body weight is transferred from one leg to the other. Unlike running, leaping requires a prolonged air phase with greater vertical height and more horizontal distance covered [6]. Early attempts at leaping typically resemble modestly exaggerated running movements. There is an inability to propel the body upward or for greater horizontal distances [8]. The arms are not used for generating force, but rather for maintaining balance. Mature leaping includes forceful extension of the support leg to maximize horizontal and vertical distances, and the arms are now coordinated and assist in force development [6].

It is important to note that an increase in chronological age does not guarantee mature jumping or leaping patterns, as adolescents and adults have been found to display immature or ineffective mechanical characteristics [6]. These can range from preparatory, takeoff, and landing inefficiencies. Therefore, coaches, teachers, and performance professionals should not assume that movement skills have been mastered simply due to chronological age. Appropriate strength and conditioning programs can help with these basic movements.

Plyometric exercises alone can improve jumping ability [9–12]. Research has shown that improvements of 12.7 % in takeoff velocity accounted for 71 % of the observed improvement in jumping performance [13]. This highlights the importance of instruction for takeoff technique and the ability to take off with maximal velocity. Therefore, landing and jumping mechanics should be viewed as separate motor skills and trained independently in the tennis athlete [6].

The combination of resistance and plyometric training caused greater improvements in vertical jump (i.e., power output) ability than either training modality alone [14]. Other research has provided indirect support for this notion by reporting that neither resistance training nor plyometric exercises alone can provide a stimulus any greater than the other when targeting performance enhancement [12]. It is important to understand that young athletes cannot increase power simply by becoming stronger and that utilizing any increase in strength at appropriate speeds is the key factor for performance enhancement [15]. This information is very relevant for strength and conditioning for young tennis players as it highlights the need to focus on strength, speed, and power development to optimize training adaptations.

Foot contacts and distance covered are the most common methods for determining plyometric volume. However, limited support exists for defined numbers of foot contacts. Studies examining the effects of plyometrics on performance have used between 30 and 200 jumps per day [9, 12, 14, 16–20]. The volume of work should be based on the intent of the session (i.e., performance versus learning), the intensity of the drills (i.e., high versus low), the training age of the athlete (i.e., inexperienced versus advanced), and other variables, including the needs of the athlete, how they play tennis (i.e., game style), and other trainings that they do (i.e., other sports) [6]. The challenge with training the competitive tennis athlete is that most players already train with excessive volume, and adding 50–200 extra high-velocity ground contacts via plyometrics may not provide the intended benefit. Power production requires a "fresh" or "rested" neuromuscular system. Therefore, low-volume plyometrics are recommended as compared to higher volume plyometrics.

The number of plyometric training sessions performed weekly will be determined by many factors. Most of the literature suggests that 2–3 days per week may be optimal for improving performance during training blocks [9, 12, 14, 16–20]. The frequency of plyometric sessions will be dictated by the need for recovery, training versus competition cycles, and how each individual will respond to the training stimulus.

Developmental Sequence of Running

Most individuals attempt to start running around 2–3 years of age or approximately 6–7 months after a child learns how to walk [7, 8]. By observing these movements in young children, this begins with a very brief flight phase with a limited range of motion in the legs. This results in a shortened stride length compared to a more mature child. In addition, the thighs and arms swing away from the body, most likely acting to help stabilize and balance the body during the flight and support phases [7]. Also to aid in balance, the stance is often wide. As children mature, they develop movement patterns that are more efficient and powerful. For example, maturity will bring about an increase in muscle mass and strength, which will provide more ground force and increase stride length [6]. Other changes in sprint mechanics include full leg extension, keeping the actions of the extremities in the anterior-posterior plane, and maintaining bent elbows [7]. However, the earlier efficient technique can be provided through guided learning techniques, the more advanced a young athlete will develop their running and movement skills.

Agility

Changes in direction occur in nearly every point in tennis and are one of the most important physical skills needed to be a successful tennis player at any level. Agility includes deceleration followed immediately by reacceleration of the entire body or individual body segment(s) [6, 21]. Agility has been described as an efficient, coordinated movement in multiple planes performed at multiple velocities [22, 23]. Although agility has been shown to be an independent athletic attribute [24], additional qualities are considered important, including dynamic balance, spatial awareness, rhythm, and visual processing [25].

In the young tennis player, the development of agility requires appropriate movement patterns and the ability to integrate locomotor skills efficiently (e.g., running, jumping) with proprioceptive awareness. As children learn to walk fast and run (at 1.5–3 years of age), they make attempts to be elusive and change direction when being chased. Their movement efficiency is often poor, however, and associated with awkward arm motion, overall unbalanced posture, and a general lack of timing and coordination. At the younger ages (prepuberty) kids should perform a large variety of general movement patterns in an effort to develop a foundation of motor skills. This could include arm and leg movements in a stationary position, rhythmic jumps in place, or locomotor drills that incorporate spatial orientation. Children before and during puberty need to become highly proficient with general drills with minimal flaws before advancing to more complex movements and especially before any type of external resistance like weight, bands, sleds, etc. Adding resistance too early to an athlete will change the movement mechanics and have a negative effect on mechanics.

Young athletes will be able to move more quickly as they mature and finish puberty. For reasons of safety and injury prevention, however, they should initially perform drills at submaximal speeds. In addition, drills should not yet include sharp changes in direction, but rather involve rounded patterns. Drills that include sharp changes in direction performed at high running speeds are unlikely to benefit agility development, especially when mastery has not yet been achieved [26, 27].

More complexity and specificity are the focus of a progressive agility training. The same drill can be made more difficult simply by using different visual and proprioceptive conditions, including a partner, or implementing an area or time restriction. Once mastery of skills has been achieved, athletes should perform nearly all of the drills at high speeds, as slower movements have been shown to alter muscle activation patterns [28]. If an athlete wants to move fast, they need to train fast. However, if muscle mechanics are compromised due to muscle imbalances or technique issues, then these areas should be improved in supplemental exercises at slower speeds or more controlled environments to ensure mastery. An example may be an athlete who struggles to change direction effectively after hitting a wide backhand ground stroke, has weak gluteus medius strength, and should therefore focus on developing gluteus medius strength in the gym while still working on agility movements close to (or at) match speed. An example would be for this athlete to perform monster walks (see Figure and Table 4.11).

Coordination and Balance

Coordination is the ability to control the movement of the body in cooperation with the body's sensory functions [29]. For example, catching a ball requires a combination of catching using your hands, eyes to visually see the ball, and then the sensory system to send the appropriate signal from the visual stimulus to the contraction of the hand to catch the ball. *Balance* is the ability to maintain equilibrium when stationary or moving (i.e., not to fall over) through the coordinated actions of our sensory functions (eyes, ears, and the proprioceptive organs in our joints) [29]. *Static balance* is the ability to retain the center of mass above the base of support in a stationary position [29]. *Dynamic balance* is the ability to maintain balance with body movement [29]. By adding movements and exercises that cause the athlete to experience different stimuli and different movement patterns at a young age, these dimensions will be developed at a faster pace at a younger age.

Strength

Training for strength is an important aspect of any athlete's physical development. Much misunderstanding and misinformation have been spread about strength training in young athletes. Below is the latest evidence-based stance on strength training in young athletes. Over the past decade the major medical and strength and conditioning associations (American Academy of Pediatrics, National Strength and Conditioning Association, and International Tennis Performance Association, among others) have come out with position statements supporting the benefits and limited risks associated with strength training in young athletes [30–32]. Below are some of the guidelines recommended to aid in successful implementation of strength training in the young athlete:

- Provide qualified instruction and supervision.
- A properly designed and supervised resistance training program is relatively safe for youth.
- A properly designed and supervised resistance training program can enhance the muscular strength and power of youth.
- A properly designed and supervised resistance training program can improve the cardiovascular risk profile of youth.
- A properly designed and supervised resistance training program can improve motor skill performance and may contribute to enhanced sports performance of youth.
- A properly designed and supervised resistance training program can increase a young athlete's resistance to sports-related injuries.
- A properly designed and supervised resistance training program can help improve the psychosocial well-being of youth.
- A properly designed and supervised resistance training program can help promote and develop exercise habits during childhood and adolescence.

Due to the large volumes of tennis practice (it is not uncommon for prepuberty tennis players to play tennis 20–25 h per week), many young tennis players struggle to reach optimum athletic development. Below are a few points and pitfalls that need to be considered when designing a fully integrated strength and conditioning program [31]:

- Young tennis players rarely spend enough time solidifying fundamentals.
- Structured formal competition-to-training ratios are too high, particularly in the early years.
- Young players are often training using similar principles, training volumes, and movement requirements as adults. This is usually inappropriate and more age- and development-specific training is appropriate.
- Young players often follow adult competition schedules.
- Too much focus on outcome goals (winning/results) and not enough focus on performance goals (task/skill development) during a tennis player's developmental years.

- Chronological age, rather than biological and training age, influences coaching and selection decisions as well as training volumes and intensities. Greater and more accurate results are achieved if developmental stage and training age are used.
- Critical periods/windows of opportunities are underutilized.
- Poorly planned programs (coaching, physical and mental) between 6 and 16 result in many athletes never reaching their genetic potential.
- If possible try not to group prepubertal athletes with postpubertal athletes, regardless of the chronological age.
- Avoid using conditioning drills as punishment. This trains the athlete to associate these drills with punishment.

Power

Power production is truly the objective with a structured tennis-specific strength and conditioning program from a performance perspective. The objective of training off-court is to improve on-court performance. Improving movement efficiency, ground reaction forces (GRF), and power is the objective to move quicker on the court. From a stroke production perspective, the goal is to increase racket head speed which is accomplished through greater power production through the successful and efficient transfer of energy from the ground up through the kinetic chain and out into the racket and ball. Studies have shown that young tennis athletes do not have as good a power production in traditional athletic assessments (vertical, jump, etc.) as other young athletes [33]. Power-focused training needs to be prioritized via the improvement of the two major aspects involved in power training – strength and speed development [34].

Flexibility

Static flexibility is when the muscle is stretched and held at a certain length with no movement [35]. Think of touching your toes and holding this stretch for 30 s. The best time to perform these exercises is after tennis practice or competition and in the evenings at home [35]. Most stretches should be held for 30 s and can be repeated two to four times depending on the level of the athlete and time available [35, 36]. Most young tennis players do not spend enough time on improving flexibility, and we know that at certain joints, for example, the glenohumeral joint, consistent tennis play will result in a decrease in range of motion [37–39].

Dynamic flexibility is when the muscle is stretched under a controlled movement pattern [35]. The muscle changes shape under a controlled lengthening and shortening process and is not performed in a jerky (or ballistic) fashion. The benefit of dynamic flexibility is that force is being produced and balance and coordination is required; research has shown that this form of flexibility is more beneficial before tennis practice or competition. It is highly recommended that dynamic flexibility be performed before tennis or physical training as opposed to static flexibility exercises [40–46]. These exercises can be accomplished on a tennis court, and the distance used for each exercises can be between the two double lines on the tennis court (36 ft). This roughly equates to approximately 10 repetitions per movement. Depending on the age and stage of development of the athlete, longer periods may be beneficial. For many elite junior players, a good dynamic warm-up will take 20–30 min working from slow controlled movements to more explosive movements that mimic the movement patterns seen on the tennis court. However, an effective dynamic warm-up can be performed in 10 min with the appropriate focus.

Exercise Selection for Strength Training in the Young Tennis Player

Upper body exercises need to be incorporated into the tennis athlete's routine. At the younger ages the purpose of upper body work is to increase muscular endurance and flexibility more than how much weight is actually lifted. The goal is to improve technique and offset any current or potential future muscle imbalances that may be created due to the large amount of hours spent on the tennis court. The main aspect of the upper body of major focus is the shoulder region. A large body of literature exists on the tennis shoulder and surrounding area, and this needs to be a major area of focus of exercises for the upper body [47–51].

Core/torso exercises are paramount to success for the tennis athlete. To effectively utilize the kinetic chain and transfer of energy, core control and stability is important [52, 53]. It is very important for both performance improvement and also to reduce the chance of injuries. The core region links the lower body with the upper body, and if the muscles of the core region are not trained effectively, it directly relates to how well a young tennis athlete can perform on the court. It is also very important to help reduce the chance of injury by improving the stability of the smaller muscles of the core region.

Lower body exercises, focused on injury prevention, are very important during a junior tennis career. If the muscles and joints in the lower body are not strong and stable, it may result in problems up through the core region and into the upper body [51, 54]. Many upper body injuries are the result of weakness in the lower body and core region, and spending appropriate time developing strength and stability in the lower body helps the young athlete progress more successfully throughout the tennis journey

Sample Exercise for the Young Tennis Player

Flexibility

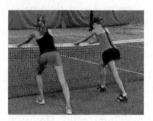

Table 4.1 Fence calf stretch [55]

Fence calf stretch [55]	
Technique	Push both hands against a solid wall (or fence) while bending the right leg (front leg) and straightening the left leg (back leg)
	Hold the stretch for 30 s and repeat using the opposite leg
Coaching cues	Maintain good body position while trying to maintain heel contact with the ground

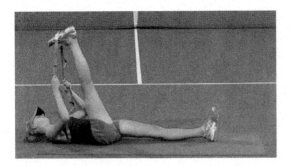

Table 4.2 Lying hamstring stretch [55]

Lying hamstring stretch [55]	
Technique	Lie supine (back on the ground) and loop a towel/rope or stretching strap around the right foot
	Keeping the leg straight and the left leg on the floor, bring the thigh closer to the body via pulling on the towel/rope/stretch strap
	Hold the stretch for 30 s and repeat
Coaching cues	Keep lower back straight with neutral spine
Variations	Knees can be straight or bent. The straight leg technique focuses on the hamstring group and the popliteus (a big word to describe a small muscle behind the knee), whereas the knee bent variation focuses on belly of the hamstring

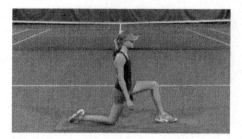

Table 4.3 Kneeling hip flexor stretch [55]

Kneeling hip flexor stretch [55]	
Technique	Start this stretch in a lunge position, with the left foot forward and the right knee on the ground (put a towel or yoga mat under the right knee on the ground)
	Maintain good posture in the upper body (shoulders back, head and back straight) and gradually move the athlete's center of mass forward and downward so the hips drop slightly toward the floor
	The stretch will be felt in the front of the right hip. Hold the stretch for 30 s and repeat
Coaching cues	Squeeze shoulder blades together while maintaining a neutral spine and eyes forward
Variations	An advanced variation involves the same position, but grasping the back foot and pulling the foot upward toward the hamstring. This increases the stretch and also develops balance and coordination

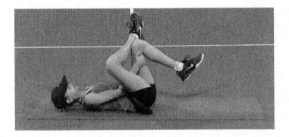

Table 4.4 Piriformis stretch [55]

Piriformis stretch [55]	
Technique	Start this stretch lying supine (on the back) on the ground (or on a mat) and cross the right ankle over the left knee while bending the left knee
	Grasp behind the left knee with both hands and pull toward the chest
	The stretch will be felt deep in the right hip/buttock. Hold the stretch for 30 s and repeat on the opposite leg
Coaching cues	Push pelvis into the floor and keep increasing the stretch
Variations	An advanced variation involves the same position, but extending the left leg (in example above), which also stretches the hamstring simultaneously

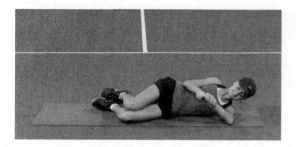

Table 4.5 Sleeper stretch

Sleeper stretch	
Technique	Lying on the left side of the body, flex the athlete's left elbow at 90° and position the left arm so that it is perpendicular to the upper body. The left hand should point to the ceiling
	With the right hand, slowly and gently push the left forearm downward toward the floor
	Hold the stretch for 30 s and repeat on the opposite arm
Coaching cues	Maintain arm position while slowly increasing the stretch and keeping the scapula stable

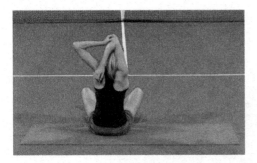

Table 4.6 Triceps stretch [55]

Triceps stretch [55]	
Technique	Reach the right hand behind the head by bending the elbow and pointing the right fingers down toward the ground
	With the left hand slowly push down against the right triceps to increase the stretch
	Gradually increase the stretch hold for 30 s
	Repeat this same movement on the opposite arm
Coaching cues	Maintain good body position by keeping the shoulders back and the back straight with a neutral spine position

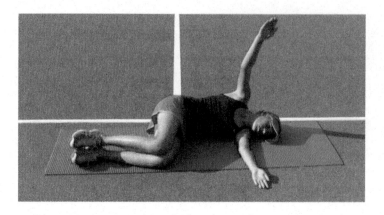

Table 4.7 Open book thoracic rotation [55]

Open book thoracic rotation [55]	
Exercise setup	N/A
Exercise technique	The athlete lies on his/her side (left side first) with knees and hips bent at approximately 90°
	Reaching the right arm (top arm) toward the ceiling while following the hand with the athlete's eyes. The movement occurs through the thoracic spine (not the shoulder)
	As the athlete holds the arm at the top of the movement, he/she takes 3–4 deep breaths and then moves the arm further toward the floor increasing thoracic rotation
	Slowly return to the start position and perform this movement for the appropriate number of repetitions (6–20) and repeat on the opposite side of the body
Coaching cues	A coaching cue for the athlete is to get the sternum to face the ceiling while the athlete keeps the arm in line with the sternum
	Variations: this movement can be performed using different breathing patterns and ranges of motion based on the flexibility and stability of the individual athlete

Lower Body Strength

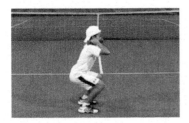

Table 4.8 Front squat – dumbbell [55]

Front squat – dumbbell [55]	
Exercise setup	Dumbbell
Exercise technique	The athlete grasps the dumbbells in both hands with feet shoulder width (or slightly further apart) with toes pointed forward or slightly out
	From an upright standing position, slowly bend the knees, and the athlete pushes the body weight through his/her heels. Keep the back straight and lower the body until the thighs are parallel to the floor (or sometimes even lower than parallel for advanced athletes)
	From the bottom of the movement, extend the knees and return to the starting position
	Repeat this same movement for the appropriate number of repetitions (1–20)
Coaching cues	A coaching cue for the athlete is to keep a strong core and good posture during the entire movement
	*Ensure that the knees do not buckle and that each knee is aligned over the second toe of the foot at the bottom of the movement
	Variations: the depth and speed of movement can be altered to accomplish the appropriate goals
Coaching cues	A coaching cue for the athlete is to keep a strong core and good posture during the entire movement. Relax the trapezius muscles while focusing on contracting the rhomboids and posterior deltoids
	Variations: this exercise can be performed using different feet positions and hand positions to stress different muscles

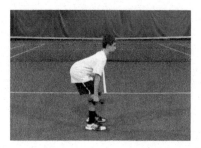

Table 4.9 Romanian dead lift – dumbbell [55]

Romanian dead lift – dumbbell [55]	
Exercise setup	Dumbbells
Exercise technique	The athlete stands with the feet shoulder width apart with the knees slightly bent (similar to an athletic position)
	While holding the dumbbells (one in each hand) in front of the body, arms down in front of the thighs resting the weight on the mid-thigh just above the knee. The athlete slowly lowers the weight to the middle of the shin by hinging at the hips. The athlete's glutes should go back and up while maintaining a subtle anterior pelvic tilt
	Return the weight back to the starting position by extending the hips and waist until the athlete returns to an upright position with the shoulders back
	Repeat this same movement for the appropriate number of repetitions
Coaching cues	A coaching cue for the athlete is to keep a strong core and good posture during the entire movement
	Variations: depth and speed may be altered depending on the goals of the athlete

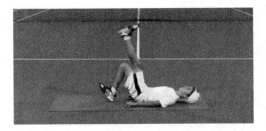

Table 4.10 Glute bridge series (hamstring buck) [55]

Glute bridge series (hamstring buck) [55]	
Exercise setup	Floor
Exercise technique	The athlete lies on his/her back with the right knee bent at approximately 45° and the right heel pressing against the floor, so that the right toe points toward the sky. The left leg will be extended straight in the air
	The athlete raises his/her hips and lower back from the ground by pushing weight through the right heel (the hands are positioned flat on the ground)
	At the top of the movement, hold the position for two seconds and then lower to the starting position
	Perform this same movement for the appropriate number of repetitions (6–20) and then repeat on the opposing leg
Coaching cues	A coaching cue for the athlete is to push through the heel and keep a straight line between the knee and the shoulders

	Variations: the exercise described above is the first in a series of more difficult movements aimed at developing functional hamstring, glute, and lower back strength and muscular endurance. By altering the hand position (crossed arms across the athlete's chest), it increases the difficulty:
	Physioball hamstring buck
	    Performed using the same movement, but the left heel is on the physioball instead of the floor
	Medicine ball hamstring buck
	    Performed using the same movement, but the left heel is on the medicine ball instead of the floor

Variation	A coaching cue for the athlete is to keep a strong core and good posture during the entire movement. Focus on transversus abdominis and multifidus control
	Variations: this exercise can be performed using a cable pulley or weight stack machine as well

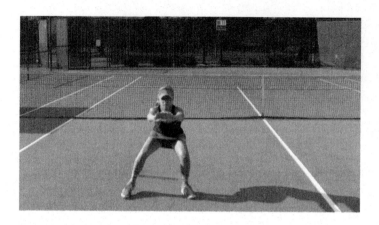

Table 4.11 Lateral monster walk [55]

Lateral monster walk [55]	
Exercise setup	Thin elastic tubing
Exercise technique	The athlete places a thin elastic band around the calves and assumes an athletic position
	From a low starting position (with thighs parallel to the ground and the knees are bent approximately 90°), the athlete takes a small step to the right using the right leg, followed by a small step with the left leg to the right returning the body to the starting position
	Perform the appropriate number of steps to the right (6–20) and then repeat for the same number of repetitions to the left
Coaching cues	A coaching cue for the athlete is to activate the gluteus medius muscles in both legs while maintaining an erect core posture
	Variations: this movement can be performed using different movement patterns (forward, backward, diagonal, lateral, etc.)

Upper Body

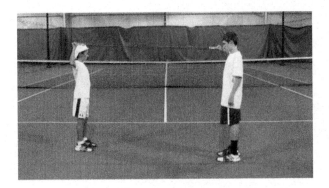

Table 4.12 90°/90° external shoulder rotation [55]

90°/90° external shoulder rotation [55]	
Exercise setup	Elastic tubing
Exercise technique	The athlete grasps the tubing with the right hand (thumb up) and while standing erect with a 90° angle at the shoulder and a 90° angle at the elbow while facing the tubing attachment
	From this starting position the athlete will externally rotate the shoulder against the tubing resistance. The forearm starts parallel to the floor and becomes perpendicular to the floor at the top of the movement. Hold near the end range of motion for approximately two seconds
	Slowly return to the starting position and repeat for the appropriate number of repetitions (8–15)
	Repeat this movement for the opposite hand
Coaching cues	A coaching cue for the athlete is to relax the trapezius muscles while contracting the rhomboids and external shoulder rotators focusing on scapula control
	Variations: this drill can be performed while also standing on one leg to increase the requirements of the stabilizing muscles of the core and lower body to be more engaged

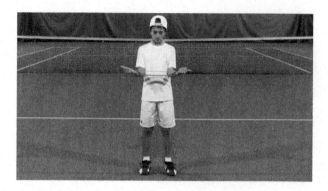

Table 4.13 Tubing scapula retraction (external rotation) [55]

Tubing scapula retraction (external rotation) [55]	
Exercise setup	Elastic tubing
Exercise technique	The athlete grasps a small amount of elastic tubing in both hands and slowly externally rotates both shoulders simultaneously while retracting both shoulder blades
	Return back to the starting position and perform this movement for the appropriate number of repetitions (10–15) to develop muscular endurance
Variation	A coaching cue for the athlete is to squeeze shoulder blades together and maintain good scapula control during all movements
	Variations: this movement can be performed using different isometric hold positions throughout the movement

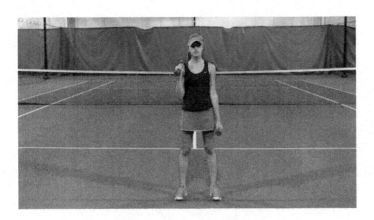

Table 4.14 Hammer curl [55]

Hammer curl [55]	
Exercise setup	Cable pulley, weight stack, resistance tubing, or dumbbell
Exercise technique	The athlete stands upright holding dumbbells (or resistance tubing) with arms extended by the sides with the thumbs pointing upward
	The athlete lifts one arm to his/her shoulder in a straight path by bending at the elbow with the thumb pointing up
	At the top of the movement, slowly lower the dumbbell back down to the starting position and repeat with the opposite arm for the required number of repetitions (6–20)
Coaching cues	A coaching cue for the athlete is to squeeze the shoulder blades together while performing the hammer curl exercise
	Variations: the hammer curl with rotation begins in the same position, but as the elbow starts to bend, the thumb rotates out via forearm supination

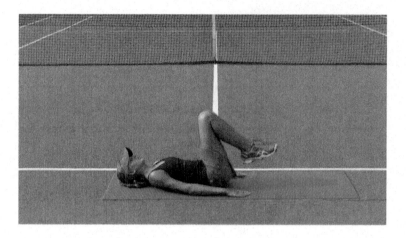

Table 4.15 Reverse crunch [55]

Reverse crunch [55]	
Exercise setup	Floor
Exercise technique	The athlete lays supine (back on ground) on the floor with hips and knees bent at 90°, with hands touching the ears
	Via contraction of the abdominal muscles, raise the pelvis from the ground via contraction of the rectus abdominis, hip flexors, and obliques
	Slowly lower the legs down to the starting position and repeat this movement for the appropriate number of repetitions (20–100)
Coaching cues	A coaching cue for the athlete is to keep a strong core and good posture during the entire movement. Focus on transversus abdominis control
	Variations: this exercise can be performed on a physioball instead of the floor to train the stabilizing muscles of the core and hip to a greater extent

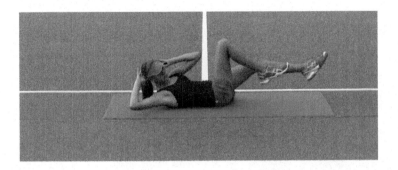

Table 4.16 Bicycles [55]

Bicycles [55]	
Exercise setup	Floor
Exercise technique	The athlete lays supine on the floor with hips and knees bent at 90°, with hands touching the ears
	Via contraction of the abdominal muscles, raise the shoulder blades from the ground via contraction of the rectus abdominis and obliques and rotate the torso moving the left elbow to the right knee
	Return back to the starting position and repeat on the opposite side
	The speed of movement can either be fast or slow, depending on the goal of the exercise within the program
	Repeat this movement for the appropriate number of repetitions (20–100)
Coaching cues	A coaching cue for the athlete is to keep a strong core and good posture during the entire movement. Focus on transversus abdominis control
	Variations: this exercise can be performed on a physioball instead of the floor to train the stabilizing muscles of the core and hip to a greater extent

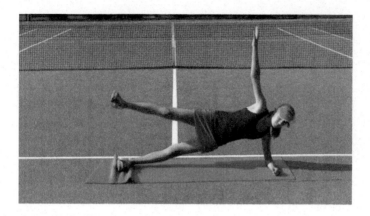

Table 4.17 Side plank/bridge variations [55]

Side plank/bridge variations [55]	
Exercise setup	Floor
Exercise technique	The athlete lays prone with elbows and forearms resting underneath the body
	The athlete then rotates onto the side with the left elbow and shoulder positioned with a 90° angle and the entire body raised from the ground except the elbow and left foot
	Via contraction of the core and hip muscles, the athlete lifts the torso and hips from the ground into a bridge position with the body weight evenly disbursed through the elbows and feet
	Hold this position while maintaining a neutral spine (flat back) for the designated period of time (30 s for the beginner athlete to 120 s for the more advanced athlete)
	The athlete will repeat the same movement on the other side of the body. *Wt may be added for the advanced athlete
Coaching cues	A coaching cue for the athlete is to keep a strong core and good posture during the entire movement. Focus on transversus abdominis control

	Variations:
	  Side plank/bridge hold (left and right)
	  Side plank/bridge hold
	  Side plank/bridge with thoracic rotations
	  Side plank/bridge with hip abduction (left and right)

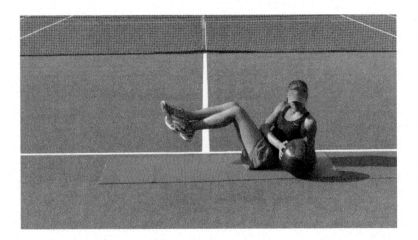

Table 4.18 Russian twist

Russian twist	
Exercise setup	Mat
	Medicine ball
Exercise technique	The athlete lies supine on a mat with the torso raised from the ground and the legs raised from the ground with hands straight out grasping a medicine ball
	The athlete slowly rotates to the right keeping the core tight via contraction of transversus abdominis and obliques
	Repeat this same movement back to the center and to the left. Perform this movement for the appropriate number of repetitions (10–50)
Coaching cues	A coaching cue for the athlete is to keep a strong core and good posture during the entire movement. Focus on core and hip position
	Variations: this exercise can be performed using a physioball which increases the difficulty of the exercise

Table 4.19 3 days a week sample strength and conditioning program for a 12 and under junior player – no experience [55]

3 days a week sample strength and conditioning program for a 12 and under junior player – no experience [55][a]				
	Reps	Sets	Resistance	Time of exercise (seconds)
Dynamic warm-up				
Walking knee-to-chest stretch	10	2	BW	30 per set
Knee-to-shoulder lateral walk	10	2	BW	30 per set
Hamstring hand walk (inchworm)	10	2	BW	30 per set
Spiderman crawl	10	2	BW	30 per set
Walking lunge	10	2	BW	30 per set
Hugs	10	2	BW	30 per set
Wipers	10	2	BW	30 per set
General strength				
MB power throws	6	3	6lbs	
Front squat – dumbbell	10	3	10lbs	
Glute bridge series	10	3	BW	
Monster walks (bands)	10	3	Green	
Low row (tubing)	10	2	Green	
90°/90° external shoulder rotation	12	2	Yellow	
Plank	1	3	BW	30 s
Side plank (each side)	1	3	BW	30 s
Bicycles	20	2	BW	
Russian twist	20	2	BW	
Static stretches				
Cross-arm stretch	3	1		30 s
Sleeper stretch	3	1		30 s
Triceps stretch	3	1		30 s
Hamstring stretch	3	1		30 s
Kneeling hip flexor stretch	3	1		30 s
Figure 4 stretch	3	1		30 s

[a]This is a strength- and power-focused example. Coordination, balance, agility, speed, and endurance training should also be performed during tennis practice and other sessions throughout the week

Table 4.20 3 days a week sample strength and conditioning program for a 16 and under junior player – minimal experience [55]

3 days a week sample strength and conditioning program for a 16 and under junior player – minimal experience [55][a]	Reps	Sets	Resistance[b]	Time of exercise (seconds)
Dynamic warm-up				
Walking knee-to-chest stretch	15	2		60 per set
Walking quad stretch	15	2		60 per set
Knee-to-shoulder lateral walk	15	2		60 per set
Hamstring hand walk (inchworm)	15	2		60 per set
Spiderman crawl	15	2		60 per set
Walking lunge	15	2		60 per set
Hugs	15	2		60 per set
Wipers	15	2		60 per set
General strength and power program				
Jump shrug	4	4		Explosive
MB granny toss	6	3		Explosive
1-leg countermovement jumps	4	5		Explosive
DB front squat	12	3		
Romanian dead lift – dumbbell	12	3		
Monster walk	20	2		
DB single-arm bench press	10	3		
External shoulder rotation – tubing	12	3		
90°/90° external shoulder rotation	12	3		
Plank	1	3	BW	30 per set
Side plank (each side)	1	3	BW	30 per set
Bicycles	20	2	BW	
Russian twist	20	2	BW	
Dead bug	25	2		
Static stretching				
Cross-arm stretch	3	1		30 per rep
Sleeper stretch	3	1		30 per rep
Triceps stretch	3	1		30 per rep
Hamstring stretch	3	1		30 per rep
Kneeling hip flexor stretch	3	1		30 per rep
Figure 4 stretch	3	1		30 per rep
Sleeper stretch	4	1		30 per rep
Triceps stretch	4	1		30 per rep

[a]This is a strength- and power-focused example. Coordination, balance, agility, speed, and endurance training should also be performed during tennis practice and other sessions throughout the week

[b]Due to the variability in age and stage of development and gender differences in this age group, resistance needs to be adjusted to fit the level of the athlete

References

1. Kibler WB, Safran M. Tennis injuries. In: Caine D, Maffuli N, editors. Epidemiology of pediatric sports injuries – individual sports. Basel: Karger; 2005. p. 120–37.
2. Hutchinson MR, Laprade RF, Burnett QM, Moss R, Terpstra J. Injury surveillance at the USTA boys' tennis championships: a 6-yr study. Med Sci Sports Exerc. 1995;27(6):826–30.
3. Reece LA, Fricker PA, Maguire KF. Injuries to elite young tennis players at the Australian institute of sport. Aust J Sci Med Sports. 1986;18:11–5.
4. Winge S, Jorgenson U, Nielson L. Epidemiology of injuries in Danish championship tennis. Int J Sports Med. 1989;10:368–71.
5. Kovacs MS, Ellenbecker TS, Kibler WB, Roetert EP. Demographic data and injury trends in American national junior tennis players. J Strength Cond Res. 2012;26(1):S62.
6. Kovacs M. Plyometric, speed and agility exercise prescription. In: Chandler TJ, Brown LE, editors. Conditioning for strength and human performance. 2nd ed. Philadelphia: Lippincott, Williams & Wilkins; 2012. p. 383–420.
7. Haywood KM, Getchell N. Life span motor development. 3rd ed. Champaign: Human Kinetics; 2001.
8. Gallahue DL, John CO. Understanding motor development. 6th ed. New York: McGraw-Hill; 2006.
9. Brown ME, Mayhew JL, Boleach LW. Effect of plyometric training on vertical jump performance in high school basketball players. J Sports Med Phys Fit. 1986;26:1–4.
10. Fatouros IG, Jamurtas AZ, Leontsini D, et al. Evaluation of plyometric exercise training, weight training, and their combination on vertical jumping performance and leg strength. J Strength Cond Res. 2000;14:470–6.
11. Luebbers PE, Potteiger JA, Hulver MW, et al. Effects of plyometric training and recovery on vertical jump performance and anaerobic power. J Strength Cond Res. 2003;17:704–9.
12. Wilson GJ, Murphy AJ, Giorgi A. Weight and plyometric training: effects on eccentric and concentric force production. Can J Appl Physiol. 1996;21:301–15.
13. Ashby BM, Heegaard JH. Role of arm motion in the standing long jump. J Biomech. 2002;35:1631–7.
14. Adams K, O'Shea J, O'Shea K, et al. The effect of six weeks of squat, plyometric, and squat-plyometric training on power production. J Appl Sports Sci Res. 1992;6:36–41.
15. Bobbert MF, Van Soest AJ. Effects of muscle strengthening on vertical jump height: a simulation study. Med Sci Sports Exerc. 1994;26:1012–20.
16. Clutch M, Wilton M. The effect of depth jumps and weight training on leg strength and vertical jump. Res Q Exerc Sport. 1983;54:5–10.
17. Diallo O, Dore E, Duche P, et al. Effects of plyometric training followed by a reduced training programme on physical performance in prepubescent soccer players. J Sports Med Phys Fit. 2001;41:342–8.
18. Gehri DJ, Ricard MD, Kleiner DM, et al. A comparison of plyometric training techniques for improving vertical jump ability and energy production. J Strength Cond Res. 1998;12:85–9.
19. Potteiger J, Lockwood R, Daub M, et al. Muscle power and fiber characteristics following 8 weeks of plyometric training. J Strength Cond Res. 1999;13:275–9.
20. Young WB, Wilson GJ, Byrne C. A comparison of drop jump training methods: effects on leg extensor strength qualities and jumping performance. Int J Sports Med. 1999;20:295–303.
21. Kovacs MS, Roetert EP, Ellenbecker TS. Efficient deceleration: the forgotten factor in tennis-specific training. Strength Cond J. 2008;30(6):58–69.
22. Drabik J. Children & sports training: how your future champions should exercise to be healthy, fit, and happy. Island Pond: Stadion; 1996.
23. Verstegen M, Marcello B. Agility and coordination. In: Foran B, editor. High performance sports conditioning. Champaign: Human Kinetics; 2001.
24. Little T, Williams AG. Specificity of acceleration, maximal speed and agility in professional soccer players. J Strength Cond Res. 2005;19(1):76–8.

25. Ellis L, Gastin P, Lawrence S, et al. Protocols for the physiological assessment of team sports players. In: Gore CJ, editor. Physiological tests for elite athletes. Champaign: Human Kinetics; 2000.
26. Besier TF, Lloyd DG, Ackland TR, et al. Anticipatory effects on knee joint loading during running and cutting maneuvers. Med Sci Sports Exerc. 2001;33:1176–81.
27. Rand MK, Ohtsuki T. EMG analysis of lower limb muscles in humans during quick change in running directions. Gait Posture. 2000;12:169–83.
28. Neptune RR, Wright IC, van der Bogert AJ. Muscle coordination and function during cutting movements. Med Sci Sports Exerc. 1999;31:294–302.
29. Davids K, Renshaw I, Glazier P. Movement models from sports reveal fundamental insights into coordination processes. Exe Sport Sci Rev. 2005;33(1):36–42.
30. Faigenbaum AD, Kraemer WJ, Blimkie CJR, Jeffreys I, Micheli LJ, Nitka M, et al. Youth resistance training: updated position statement paper from the National Strength and Conditioning Association. J Strength Cond Res. 2009;23(5):S60–79.
31. ITPA. Certified Tennis Performance Specialist (CTPS) workbook and study guide. Atlanta: International Tennis Performance Association; 2012.
32. CoSMaF AAP. Strength training by children and adolescents. Pediatrics. 2008;121(4):835–40.
33. Bencke J, Damsgaard R, Saekmose A, Jorgensen P, Jorgensen K, Klausen K. Anaerobic power and muscle strength characteristics of 11 years old elite and non-elite boys and girls from gymnastics, team handball, tennis and swimming. Scand J Med Sci Sports. 2002;12(3):171–8.
34. Kovacs M, Chandler WB, Chandler TJ. Tennis training: enhancing on-court performance. Vista: Racquet Tech Publishing; 2007.
35. Kovacs M. Dynamic stretching: the revolutionary new warm-up method to improve power, performance and range of motion. Berkeley: Ulysses Press; 2010.
36. Roetert EP, Ellenbecker TS. Complete conditioning for tennis. 2nd ed. Champaign: Human Kinetics; 2007.
37. Kibler WB, Chandler TJ. Range of motion in junior tennis players participating in an injury risk modification program. J Sci Med Sport. 2003;6(1):51–62.
38. Kibler WB, Chandler TJ, Livingston BP, Roetert EP. Shoulder range of motion in elite tennis players: effect of age and years of tournament play. Am J Sports Med. 1996;24(3):279–85.
39. Kovacs MS, Ellenbecker TS, Kibler WB, editors. Tennis recovery: a comprehensive review of the research. Boca Raton: USTA; 2009.
40. Fowles JR, Sale DG, MacDougall JD. Reduced strength after passive stretch of the human plantar flexors. J Appl Physiol. 2000;89(3):1179–88.
41. DeVries HA. The "looseness" factor in speed and O^2 consumption of an anaerobic 100-yard dash. Res Q. 1963;34(3):305–13.
42. Kokkonen J, Nelson AG, Cornwell A. Acute muscle stretching inhibits maximal strength performance. Res Q Exerc Sport. 1998;69:411–5.
43. Nelson AG, Guillory IK, Cornwell A, Kokkonen J. Inhibition of maximal voluntary isokinetic torque production following stretching is velocity specific. J Strength Cond Res. 2001;15(2):241–6.
44. Nelson AG, Kokkonen J. Acute ballistic muscle stretching inhibits maximal strength performance. Res Q Exerc Sport. 2001;72(4):415–9.
45. Avela J, Kyröläinen H, Komi PV. Altered reflex sensitivity after repeated and prolonged passive muscle stretching. J Appl Physiol. 1999;86(4):1283–91.
46. Fletcher IM, Jones B. The effect of different warm-up stretch protocols on 20-m sprint performance in trained rugby union players. J Strength Cond Res. 2004;18(4):885–8.
47. Ellenbecker TS. Shoulder internal and external rotation strength and range of motion in highly skilled tennis players. Isokinetics Exe Sci. 1992;2:1–8.
48. Ellenbecker TS, Pluim B, Vivier S, Sniteman C. Common injuries in tennis players: exercises to address muscular imbalances and reduce injury risk. Strength Cond J. 2009;31(4):50–8.
49. Ellenbecker TS, Roetert EP. Effects of a 4-month season on glenohumeral joint rotational strength and range of motion in female collegiate tennis players. J Strength Cond Res. 2002;16(1):92–6.

50. Ellenbecker TS, Roetert EP, Baillie DS, Davies GJ, Brown SW. Glenohumeral joint total rota-
    tion range of motion in elite tennis players and baseball pitchers. Med Sci Sports Exerc.
    2002;34(12):2052–6.
51. Ellenbecker TS, Roetert EP, Kibler WB, Kovacs MS. Applied biomechanics of tennis. In:
    Magee D, Manske RC, Zachazewski J, editors. Athletic and sports issues in musculoskeletal
    rehabilitation. St. Louis: Saunders; 2010.
52. Hirashima M, Yamane K, Nakamura Y, Ohtsuki T. Kinetic chain of overarm throwing in terms
    of joint rotations revealed by induced acceleration analysis. J Biomech. 2008;41(13):
    2874–83.
53. Roetert EP, Groppel JL. Mastering the kinetic chain. In: Roetert EP, Groppel JL, editors. World
    class tennis technique. Champaign: Human Kinetics; 2001. p. 99–113.
54. Kibler WB. The 4000-watt tennis player: power development for tennis. Med Sci Tennis.
    2009;14(1):5–8.
55. iTPA. The parent's guide to basic injury prevention for the junior tennis player. Atlanta:
    International Tennis Performance Association; 2013.

Chapter 5
Periodization and Recovery in the Young Tennis Athlete

Satoshi Ochi and Mark S. Kovacs

Periodization Concepts

Although traditional linear periodization concepts may not apply easily for a tennis player because of a long season, inability to estimate effectively wins and losses each week at tournaments, high training volumes, and a shifting schedule as ranking improves/decreases results in the ability to play in different levels of tournaments. It is important to understand basic concepts of periodization and program design to create an annual training plan for a young tennis athlete. Periodization is a program design strategy to utilize systematic variations in training specificity, intensity, and volume to promote long-term training and performance improvements and minimize risk of injuries and other symptoms associated with overtraining [5, 11, 25].

General Adaptation Syndrome (GAS)

The manner in which the human body reacts to any type of training stress has been described as general adaptation syndrome (GAS) [25]. When the human body experiences a new or more intense training stress, the first response is the shock or alarm phase. During this shock/alarm phase, athletes may experience soreness, stiffness, and

S. Ochi, MA, CSCS, RSCC*D, CTPS, MTPS (✉)
USTA Player Development Incorporated, 10399 Flores Drive, Boca Raton, FL 33428, USA
e-mail: Ochi@usta.com

M.S. Kovacs, PhD, FACSM, CSCS*D, CTPS, MTPS
Life Sport Science Institute and Department of Sport Health Science, Life University,
Marietta, GA, USA
e-mail: kovacs@itpa-tennis.org; http://www.itpa-tennis.org

© Springer International Publishing Switzerland 2016
A.C. Colvin, J.N. Gladstone (eds.), *The Young Tennis Player*: *Injury Prevention and Treatment*, Contemporary Pediatric and Adolescent Sports Medicine,
DOI 10.1007/978-3-319-27559-8_5

a temporary drop in performance. Next is the resistance phase, where the body adapts to the stimulus from the first stage and returns to more normal functioning. During this phase, an athlete's body is able to demonstrate its ability to withstand stress, an attribute that may continue for an extended period of time. Here, an athlete may also experience improvement in strength, speed, power, and body structure. However, if the stress lasts for an extended time, an exhaustion phase has been reached. Here one may experience some of the same symptoms felt during the alarm phase. As a result, overtraining may occur when there is no training variety throughout the programs. The periodization concept will apply adequate amounts of stress on an athlete's body over a period of time to promote optimal amounts of positive adaptations to the training and avoid risk of injury, especially overuse injuries and overtraining.

General Training Principles

Specificity The method of training an athlete in a specific manner to produce a specific adaptation or training outcome. This concept is also known as Specific Adaptation to Imposed Demands (SAID). Training must be specific to the sport of tennis, level of the athletes, biological age, and training age/experience [1, 2].

Overload To create a positive training adaptation and outcomes, training workload and intensity must be greater than the athlete is accustomed to [1, 2].

Progression If a training program is to continue producing higher levels of performance, the intensity of the training must become progressively greater. Progression, when applied properly, promotes long-term training benefits. The periodization concept will help to create proper variations of progression [1, 2].

Periodization Cycles

Macrocycle The largest division of the periodization program is typically an entire training year. It also could be less or more than 1 year. It is possible to have two macrocycles in one calendar year, or a macrocycle could last 4 years, for example, with Olympic athletes. A 1-year macrocycle is usually appropriate for a tennis player [11, 25].

Mesocycle The macrocycle consists of two or more mesocycles. Each mesocycle is usually several weeks to several months. Often times sport seasons, for example, off-season, preseason, in-season, and postseason, are used as mesocycles. However, because of a long in-season for a tennis player, it may need to have multiple mesocycles during in-season, and sometimes a season may not be the best mesocycle option [11, 25].

Microcycle Each mesocycle consists of two or more microcycles. Using each training calendar week as a microcycle is appropriate for most of the tennis athletes but could last up to 10–14 days depending on the program and training goal [11, 25].

Periodization Periods

The modern conventional periodization model has the following four periods: preparatory, first transition, competitive, and second transition. When designing a periodized program, these training periods help identify training goals and vary the training design variables.

Preparatory Period The preparatory period is usually the longest and occurs during the time of the year when the athletes do not have much tennis skill training or on-court practice and tournaments. The beginning and initial phase of the preparatory period usually uses a general preparatory phase where an athlete can spend more time on an introductory light intensity/moderate- to high-volume training, especially for beginning athletes or an athlete who has taken some time away from training. In contrast to the general preparatory phase, the specific preparatory phase consists of exercises and programs that are more specific to the athlete's goals and focus on more tennis-specific strength, acceleration, power, and agility training [11, 25].

First Transition/Pre-competition Period Between the preparatory and competitive periods, athletes benefit from higher-intensity and lower-volume training than preparatory period along with more tennis-specific agility, footwork, movement, acceleration, strength, and power. This period is called first transition or pre-competition phase [11, 25].

Competitive Period Tennis involves year-round competition at both the junior and professional level. This makes it difficult to apply traditional periodization programs to tennis athletes because most of the periodization concepts are designed to apply to sports that have a shorter competitive season. The collegiate tennis season in the USA allows for more traditional periodization programs since the main competition period is about 4 months long and ends with championship tournaments. During the competitive period, there are two major phases, maintenance phase and peaking phase. Manipulating moderate intensity with moderate volume for the maintenance phase is usually appropriate for a tennis athlete. On-court skill and tennis practice is the priority during this period so that it is important to modify off-court training to maximize on-court time when it is necessary [11]. The peaking phase is used for the major competitions. For professional players it could be four grand slams, and for junior players (depends on the level of players), it could be regional, national, or some major international tournaments. Unlike other sports that usually have end of the season championships, tennis has multiple peaking phases in one season. The well-designed peaking phase program promotes full rest and recovery for the major competitions by decreasing the volume of the training while upholding fairly high intensity.

Second Transition Period (Active Rest) After the last tournament/match of the year and until the next macrocycle's preparatory period is the second transition period or active rest. During this period, there is almost no to very minimum on-court tennis practice, and often times cross-training methods are utilized, playing other sports or different modes of training [11, 25]. It is also used for time to heal or focus on treatment for the injuries that may occur during the competitive period. Another way to use second transition or active rest is to insert a 1-week break between long phases or periods. It is often referred to as unloading or download week. This will promote optimum rest from the previous training phase and make transition to the next training phase to promote further positive adaptations to the training. It is also believed that inserting an unloading or download week helps prevent overtraining.

Application to Young Tennis Athletes

As previously mentioned the uniqueness of the tennis calendar schedule makes it difficult to apply traditional periodization concepts. Also, it is important to understand and take into consideration a young tennis player's individual characteristics, goals, and needs.

The training programs and periodization plan must follow the specificity concept. Therefore, it needs to be specific for a young tennis athlete. The major consideration is that a child is in a constant state of change and is not a miniature adult. As young children grow, they become taller and heavier, change body composition, and increase the size of various organs, along with other physiological changes [6, 21, 23]. It is important to note that each child has different rates and timing of growth and maturation. Therefore, understating and awareness of each child's status with regard to puberty is the key to develop a periodization plan for a young tennis athlete. Puberty is the period during which skeletal, sexual, and somatic changes occur, and once again its timing can vary greatly from child to child. Peak height velocity (PHV) or growth spurt occurs approximately 12 years of age in female and approximately at 14 years of age in male. Usually the first sign of puberty in girls or onset of menstruation occurs about 12–15 months after PHV [11, 21, 23]. PHV curve in boys is much steeper than in girls and on average occurs about 2 years after the first sign of puberty. PHV and puberty are oftentimes used as a guide to identify a child's development stage. For a young tennis athlete, it is important to prescribe an appropriate training mode to develop certain physical and motor skills at the right moment as well as adjusting intensity and volume for each stage of development. Chronological age for each development stage is used as a reference point since a wide variety of age differences are expected for the onset puberty and PHV. Monitoring of each child's growth closely to understand his or her biological age instead of chronological age is appropriate to identify each child's development stage. Prepuberty, puberty, and postpuberty are a simple way to describe development stage. Since each stage is very general and not very specific to athletic population, the Long-Term Athletic Development (LTAD) model has been utilized to offer a more strategic approach to the athletic development of youth. Recently, the International Tennis Performance Association (ITPA) has introduced the following Five-Set Model to Lifetime Tennis Performance Development as tennis-specific LTAD: Set 1, Active Start and Fundamentals (FUNdamentals); Set 2, Learning to Train and Training to Train; Set 3, Training to Compete; Set 4, Training to Win; and Set 5, Tennis/Fitness for Life (it will not be discussed in this chapter since the age group for the Set 5 is adulthood) [3, 7, 11, 19]. These stages are very helpful to develop periodization models for young tennis athletes specific to growth and development.

It is important for tennis coaches and parents to consider a young tennis player's long-term development as an athlete and person. Traditional periodization cycles and periods are a great way to understand and create an annual plan. However, especially for a young athlete, it is important to see a big picture and an entire tennis career as a one big macrocycle and each development stage as big mesocycles. Figure 5.1 summarizes this theory and helps to understand the periodization concept and lifetime tennis performance development. Please note, actual individual development varies and ages are approximate chronological ages.

Periodization for Each Set Model to Lifetime Tennis Performance Development

Set 1: Active Start and FUNdamental (Approximate Chronological Age, <10 Years of Age)

The main goal for Set 1 is to learn the basic physical and tennis skills in a fun environment. This is why the term "FUNdamental" is used. Ten and under tennis format helps to develop fundamental tennis skills with age and development appropriate equipment and court size. During this stage the focus should be to learn the basic physical and tennis skills in a fun environment. The periodization is not yet utilized at this stage. However, it is important to develop basic movement skills and agility, balance, and coordination (ABCs), which many early specialized tennis players do not develop properly. ABCs and fundamental movements include jumping, hopping, catching, receiving, balance, agility, feet and hand coordination, kicking, hitting, throwing, skipping, and so on. Children develop these fundamental movements from daily physical activities including the playground [3, 7, 8, 11, 24]. Also, playing different sports other than tennis will help develop fundamental movements and skills as well as possibly prevent overuse injuries and burnout [10, 20]. Therefore, it is recommended to involve different sports and not to specialize in one sport, like tennis, at this stage and possibly not until middle or late adolescence [12, 14]. Set 1 could use as general preparatory period of a child's lifelong macrocycle (Fig. 5.1).

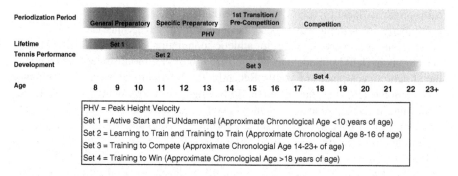

Fig. 5.1 Periodization period and lifetime tennis performance development. *PHV* peak height velocity, *Set 1* active start and FUNdamental (approximate chronological age <10 years of age), *Set 2* learning to train and training to train (approximate chronological age 8–16 of age), *Set 3* training to compete (approximate chronological Age 14–23+ of age), *Set 4* training to win (approximate chronological Age >18 years of age)

Set 2: Learning to Train and Training to Train (Approximate Chronological Age, 8–16 Years of Age)

As shown in Fig. 5.1, this stage could be considered as specific preparatory period of a child's lifelong macrocycle. The main goal for Set 2 is to solidify the fundamental skills learned during Set 1. Since the approximate chronological age for this stage could overlap with PHV and onset puberty, it is important to monitor a child's growth and use PHV as paramount reference point. It is recommended to measure a child's stature once a week to monitor and make necessary adjustments based on a child's growth stage [21]. Because of the amount of physiological changes in a child's body, it is normal to see a temporary drop in some of the skills that a child learned and developed previously. However, strong foundation and continuities of the program make easier transition and a greater possible improvement during post-puberty. Also, critical periods, known as optimum windows of opportunity, should be considered and implemented when designing a young tennis player's periodization plan during this stage so that a child has optimum development of skills and physical/athletic components [3, 8, 11, 19]:

Flexibility Optimal window for both genders is between 6 and 10 years of age. Flexibility is one of the characters that a child may lose during PHV. Therefore, it is also important to focus on flexibility training during PHV.

Agility and Quickness (Speed 1) Optimal window for boys occurs between the ages of 7 and 9 years and 6 and 8 years for girls. This is why agility and quickness along with balance and coordination (ABC) are one of the main focuses during Set 1 Active Start and FUNdamental. Agility and quickness drills should be very short-duration movements (<5 s).

Motor Skills Optimal window for motor skills is between 9 and 12 years for boys and between 8 and 11 for girls. Therefore, it is also a critical time to develop the fundamental athlete skills and tennis movements. Therefore, especially at the beginning of the Set 2 is the major skill learning stage of development.

Speed (Speed 2) For boys, optimal window occurs between the ages of 13 and 16. For girls it is between the ages of 11 and 13 years. During this periods, training should be focused on maximum speed development along with agility and quickness exercises/movements <15–20 s.

Aerobic Capacity Because the optimal window is at the onset of PHV, aerobic capacity training is suggested before athletes reach PHV. If the foundation of a child's aerobic capacity is successfully developed at an early age, it will help to make an easier transition to develop more tennis-specific endurance later. It is important to note that this optimal window of opportunity may be the same timing as a child starts having some growth-related pains, such as Osgood-Schlatter disease (knee pain), that may limit some of the activities like running. Exercise mode needs to be adjusted based on the child's condition, and proper screening and diagnosis should be done by the child's pediatrician or orthopedist.

Strength Optimal window for boys is 6–18 months after PHV and immediately after PHV (and/or at the onset of menarche) for girls. It is important to note that strength training is safe and effective at all ages. Of course, young athletes may need more attention and adjust intensity and volume accordingly. When a child can follow the direction and is coachable, he or she can participate and perform strength training exercises safely [6, 18].

An appropriate planning and periodization should be utilized for Set 2, especially later in the stage when a player participates in more tournaments per year (which is similar to the periodization plans for step 3 discussed next). At the beginning of step 2 when a child is still in transition from step 1 and working on more general overall physical and athletic development, planning and periodization should consider following general guidelines [3, 11]:

- Training vs. competition ratios should be 70–80 % training and 20–30 % competition.
- At this stage, participation in other sports is still recommended (no early specialization).
- It is important to stay active. However, a child should take more than one full day (2 days ideally) off from tennis per week.
- Weekly hours of training (tennis and other training) should be 12–17 h [9].
- Introduce recovery activities and methods for the off days from tennis (discussed later in this chapter).

- At least take 1 month off from tennis per year.

Set 3: Training to Compete (Approximate Chronological Age, 14–23 ± Years of Age)

As previously mentioned, later stages of Set 2 will overlap with this stage. This is the stage that a child starts training more as a young tennis athlete and can specialize only in tennis, especially in late adolescence [12, 14]. Therefore, this stage could be classified as a transition phase to a higher level as a tennis player. Some of the children may still be going through their PHV, especially at the beginning of this stage. Because chronological ages for this stage are very varied, training age along with the biological age (PHV) has to be considered to create periodization plans for this stage [11, 21]. Training age is how many years an athlete has been training for tennis at a competitive level. This will probably greatly affect the level of play for each tennis player. The level of play will affect the level of the tournament played and it will affect the annual plan for the athlete. For example, a 16-year-old male player who has been training competitively for tennis since 14 years old has a chronological age of 16, but his training age is only 2 years old and may not be able to compete or qualify for higher-level events yet. In contrast, the same chronological age boy who has been training tennis competitively since 10, would have a tennis training age of 6 years old and may already compete in higher-level national or international-level events. Of course, each player's biological age will affect their training plans as well, but these two athletes' periodization plans will be different. Please see sample periodization plans in Figs. 5.2 and 5.3.

Steps to Create a Periodization Plan

Step 1. Decide the number of tournaments to play and write down on the calendar.
As mentioned previously, it is very possible to play tournaments every week. It is critical to schedule the tournaments to minimize the chance of injuries and potential burnout [12–14]. The general idea of training vs. competition ratio for the Set 3 is 40–60 % training and 60–40 % competition. USTA Player Development suggests maximum of 60 matches per year at age 14 and maximum of 90 matches per year at the age 16 and older [11]. Jayanthi et al. [13] studied training and competition volumes for junior tennis players. The recommendations are as follows: (1) consider playing <2 tournaments per month to reduce injury risk and (2) consider playing <18 tournaments annually in the 18 and under division (and potentially less tournaments per year than age).

Step 2. Select tournaments that the athlete needs to be at peak.
From a player's perspective, all of the tournaments are equally important. Again, especially for young tennis athletes, they are still developing overall physical fitness levels as an athlete and tennis skills as a tennis player. It is a long process, so players and coaches need to be on the same page with respect to their goal. Because of the long season of tournaments, it is important prioritize the tournament and decide which tournament(s) to

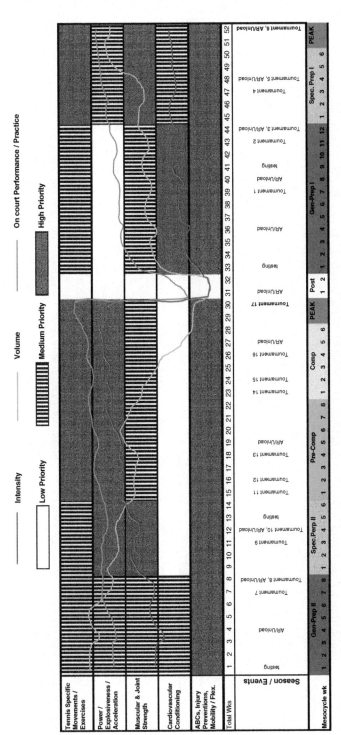

Fig. 5.2 Sample of 52 weeks periodization for 16-year-old boy with <2 years training. *AR* active rest, *Gen-Prep* general preparatory phase, *Spec. Prep* specific preparatory phase, *Comp* competitive phase, *PEAK* peaking phase, *Post* post season. 17 tournaments a year, 1st peak at end of the year holiday/new year tournament (tournament 6). 2nd (main) peak at last summer tournament (tournament 17). 1st peak is a part of preparatory phase. Low overall intensity and medium overall volume to build foundations during 1st preparatory phase (Gen. Prep I and Spec. Prep I). Throughout of the year, on court tennis practice, ABC's injury preventions, mobility and flexibility are high priorities. Try not to schedule three tournaments in a row. Use some of the tournaments as active rest or unloading week

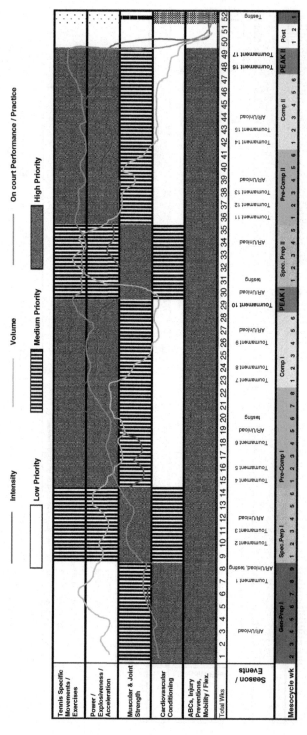

Fig. 5.3 Sample of 52 weeks periodization for 16-year-old boy with 6+ years training. *AR* active rest, *Gen-Prep* general preparatory phase, *Spec. Prep* specific preparatory phase, *Comp* competitive phase, *PEAK* peaking phase, *Post* post season. 17 tournaments a year, 1st peak at summer national tournament (tournament 10). 2nd peak at the end of the year International Jr. Tournaments (tournament 16 &17). Throughout of the year, ABC's injury preventions, mobility and flexibility are high priorities. More distinguished cycles and variations of overall intensity and volume than a player with less experience or a lower level player (Fig. 5.2). Max of three tournaments in a row

be peak at. Also, by deciding which tournament to peak at, it decides how many training cycles (periodization cycles) are per year. For most players, 2–3 peaks per year are realistic and practical [11, 24].

Step 3. Select day(s)/week(s) for rest/recovery and unload.

This is probably the most important step when creating an annual periodization plan; however, at the same time, it is probably the most forgotten step. After deciding tournament schedules, recovery days and weeks are usually assigned after each tournament. It is also important to consider building in recovery/unloading day(s) or week for each mesocycle and microcycle. For a mesocycle, the three-to-one (3:1) split is one of the popular methods to build in an unloading (also known as download) week (Fig. 5.4). With this method, after 3 weeks of training, an athlete will take a week off (unloading week). During the unloading week, normal training routine will continue; however, volume or intensity may be reduced to about half of the previous training week.

It is recommended to take off more than 1 day per week from tennis training if training over 16 h per week [13]. So each microcycle (1 week) should consist of a total of 2 days off from tennis training. One of the popular method is to take one full day off (usually on Sunday if there is no tournament) and take two half days off (Fig. 5.5).

Step 4. Assign mesocycles and decide training objectivities and goals for each mesocycle.

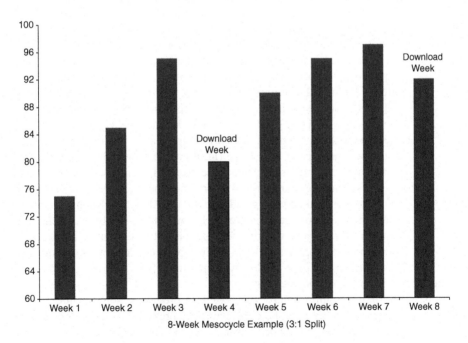

Fig. 5.4 Eight week mesocycle example (3:1 split) (Chart adapted from ITPA [11])

Monday	Tuesday	Wednesday	Thursday	Friday	Saturday	Sunday
Dynamic Warm-up	Dynamic Warm-up	Dynamic Warm-up	Dynamic Warm-up	Dynamic Warm-up	Dynamic Warm-up	
SAP	SAP	SAP	SAP	SAP	SAP	
Morning Practice						
TSE	Recovery	TSE	Recovery	TSE	Recovery	
Dynamic Warm-up	Dynamic Warm-up		Dynamic Warm-up	Dynamic Warm-up		OFF
SAP	SAP	Recovery	SAP	SAP		
Afternoon Practice			Afternoon Practice			
UL	LH		UH	LL		
Static Stretching	Static Stretching		Static Stretching	Static Stretching		

SAP	On-Court Speed Agility and Power (10-15 minutes)
TSE	Tennis Specific Endurance (30-45 minutes)
UL	Upper Body Light (Strength Training)
LH	Lower Body Heavy (Strength Training)
RECOVERY	Structured Recovery (Stretching, Foam Rolling, Ice Baths)
UH	Upper Body Heavy (Strength Training)
LL	Lower Body Light (Strength Training)

Fig. 5.5 A single week Microcycle example. *SAP* on-court speed agility and power (10–15 min). *TSE* tennis specified endurance (30–45 min). *UL* upper body light (strength training). *LH* lower body heavy (strength training). *RECOVERY* structured recovery (stretching, foam rolling, ice baths). *UH* upper body heavy (strength training). *LL* lower body light (strength training) (Chart modified and recreated from iTPA [11])

There should be an overall theme and goal for an athlete. Each mesocycle plan has more specific goal, for example, tennis-specific movement as pre-competition phase or muscle hypertrophy as off-season training. Of course, an individual development stage as a tennis player (training age) and person (biological age) will affect actual training goals and programs. As previously mentioned, two same chronological age children might have different biological or training ages.

Testing and assessment is another important aspect of periodization planning. It will give a good baseline idea for the athlete, especially at the beginning of the year or off-season to help create realistic goals. Testing should be scheduled at least twice (ideally three to four times) per year to see the athlete's progress and make necessary adjustments of the goals and programs. The beginning or end of some of the mesocycles is usually a good time to schedule testing and assessment. Also, for a young athlete, it is important to monitor their growth by measuring height and weight at least monthly (ideally weekly) because this helps to identify an athlete's growth and development stage to apply appropriate training programs and not to miss the optimal windows of opportunity [21].

Step 5. Design each microcycle program.

When designing microcycle (weekly) programs, some of the predetermining factors must be considered. As previously mentioned in step 3, recovery days should be built in. Tennis practice schedules are usually set for the week based on the court availabilities, coaches' schedules, etc. Therefore, communication with tennis coaches to discuss available days and times for off-court training is critical. As also previously mentioned, the higher the athlete's level (more tennis training), the greater the demand for off-court training, not only to improve performance but also to prevent overuse injuries [13, 17]. Also, if a child goes to a normal traditional school, the majority of the days are preoccupied with school schedules.

Once again, an athlete's training and biological ages will greatly affect actual weekly programs. Also, time of the year and mesocycle will change structure of the weekly plan. Lastly, timing of each training mode needs to be considered. For example, it makes sense to perform more power/explosive exercises at the beginning of the week when an athlete's body is fresh. Some of the non-fatigue speed, agility, and power (SAP) exercises will help to warm up an athlete's body and stimulate proper neurological pattern, so it makes sense to do these before tennis practice (Fig. 5.5).

Step 6. Review and be ready to make adjustments day by day and week by week.

Periodization is a great way to organize a young tennis player's annual and monthly plans and on- and off-court training weekly plans and provide a clear direction of a player's development pathway as a tennis player. However, it is important to recognize that the plan requires constant review and adjustments. A tournament might be scheduled for a full week. However, it will not be a week-long tournament if a player loses in an early round. There is a great different in physical fatigue levels between a 6–0, 6–0 1 h match win and a 7–6, 6–7, 7–6 over 3 h match. It will affect the recovery method and training and practice for the next day or preparation for the next match. Weather can affect practice and training schedules. A coach may plan for a tough day of practice. However, it rained and turned into a full day of fitness when a strength and conditioning coach originally planned for a light day of fitness. School and social stresses will affect an athlete's fatigue and motivation levels. The plan must be adjusted based on an athlete's day-to-day condition. As the topic of this chapter, for a young athlete, once again his or her body will change dramatically, and the plans and programs need to be adjusted consistently based on an athlete's growth and development stage [21]. And lastly, and hopefully it will not happen too often, injury will change the whole plan for the athlete if it occurs.

Set 4: Training to Win (Approximate Chronological Age, >18 Years of Age)

At this stage, majority of players are specialized in tennis and may play in college or lower-level professional events. Most of the females are fully grown physically when entering this stage. However, some of the male athletes may still be growing and may see the second set of growth spark early in this stage. College tennis has more defined seasons and more traditional conventional periodization may apply for college tennis. For the entry-level professionals, the "step-by-step periodization plan" should be utilized. The training and competition ratio will be 25 % training and 70 % competition [11]. The tournaments and match numbers may be increased from the previous stage. Because of the tournament schedules and locations, the amount of travel may increase, and this needs to be accounted for in the consideration of periodization because it creates new stress mentally and physically and it could affect training schedules, especially traveling between different time zones or internationally. The amount of tournaments and travel may create more challenging situations than previous stages to apply the periodization plan. However, it is still possible and important to create a periodization plan that fits into the athlete's schedules and needs. Women's Tennis Association (WTA) Tour's Professional Development Programmes (PDPs) provide tools and help young female professional tennis players to schedule their tournaments and training weeks to create appropriate periodization plans. As a young professional athlete (for both male and female), having specialized professionals as a support team to create an overall plan is critical at this stage [22].

Recovery

Well-designed periodization consists of systematic means of rest and recovery. When an athlete continues training without sufficient recovery, it may negatively affect their performance, lead to over training and injury,, and could end causing burnout [4, 5]. Even the best athletes in the world who compete at the Olympic Games struggle to find the fine line between pushing themselves to the limit without overstepping to the point of overtraining and negative performance. More than 25 % of all Olympians report being over trained for the Olympics [15]. However, for most young tennis players, overtraining is rarely the problem. The typical limiting factor in tennis training is inadequate recovery (known as under-recovery). There are more than 200 potential physical and psychological symptoms that are connected with overtraining and under-recovery [11]. Fatigue is one of the common terms to describe the symptoms. It is a sensation of tiredness associated with decrements in muscular and nervous system performance and function. It is a player's responsibility to listen to his/her body and look after his/her body.

Rest Days

As previously mentioned, ideally rest days of once a week and for a young tennis player twice per week may be needed [11, 17]. A rest day should include some light activities, such as socializing with friends, going to the mall, and playing another sport that is not physically as taxing. The main purpose of rest days is to give the body optimal recovery, so an athlete should avoid any activities or environment (e.g., excessive sun exposure) that could be counterproductive [4, 11].

Recovery and Nutrition

Nutrition plays a major role in recovery. Proper nutrition will help not only the recovery but also the growth of a young tennis player. The major goals of nutritional recovery include replenishing glycogen (muscle and liver energy) stores, restoring appropriate fluid and electrolyte levels, creating new muscle protein, creating other cellular components, and restoring the immune system [11]. The level and amount of play and training, training phase, growth and development stages, and some environmental factors will affect actual amount of nutrient intake. Each player should monitor and check nutritional status regularly and make sure to consume enough nutrition to recover. It is very common that a young athlete is not consuming enough calories and nutrients every day. Especially with heavy training, it is difficult to consume enough calories and nutrients from foods, and in some cases ergogenic aids or supplements are suggested. It is important to consult with a certified professional before starting any ergogenic aids or supplements, and a young athlete should never take any products on their own.

Recovery Techniques and Modalities

There are many different recovery techniques and modalities that have been used by tennis players. It is important to understand the characteristics of each method and use them with appropriate timing and amount for optimal benefits. Any techniques and modalities should not be used for the first time during the competition (unless it is an emergency). An athlete should gain experience during training and get used to the methods since some of the methods may give an athlete's body an unexpected and unpleasant effect, such as additional soreness and stiffness from a deep tissue massage. For more in-depth analysis of recovery techniques for tennis, see the review by Kovacs and Baker 2014 [16]. Below are some of the most common recovery techniques used by tennis players.

- Hydrotherapies [4]
  Some forms of hydrotherapies have been in use for several thousand years. Warm/hot bath in body temperature (34–36 °C/93–97 °F) helps in the circulatory, pulmonary, renal, and musculoskeletal system. Alternating from cool to warm water immersion can accelerate metabolic activity to help recovery. Cold water also known as ice bath is a widely used method by athletes for recovery. A range of 10–15 °C/50–59 °F for 10–15 min is recommended. Spa is one of the common warm water immersions used by athletes. However, little scientific evidence is

available and most reports are anecdotal. Saunas (hot and dry heat) are not well understood by coaches and athletes. As a result saunas can be misused by athletes and can be detrimental to health and performance if a player dehydrates or experiences a severe reduction in central drive. Because many players misuse saunas, it is not recommended for use by young athletes, and certain institutes of sport restrict the use of saunas to athletes over 15 years of age. Showering is one of the effective modalities for recovery. If done within 5–10 min after the end of the training session, it can accelerate recovery. If a pool is available, active and static stretching (5–20 min) in the pool is also beneficial.

- Sports Massage
  Massage is a popular recovery method. However, little scientific evidence is available to support claims such as improved blood flow, improved muscle strength, or significant reductions in muscle soreness. Many studies have shown benefits in psychological factors such as mood and well-being [4, 11].
- Compressive Clothing
  In recent years, compressive clothing and garments have become fashionable with athletes in the hopes of reducing injury, benefiting performance, and enhancing recovery. Reduced perception of fatigue and enhanced clearance of blood lactate and creatine kinase have been reported with compression garments compared with passive recovery [4, 11]. Although more studies are needed, a combination of hydrotherapy techniques followed by the use of compressive garments appears to be beneficial for tennis players between matches and post-training [16].
- Electronic Interventions
  Electronic stimulation is available in different forms. When it is used for recovery purposes, it can help by increasing muscle blood flow which helps accelerate muscle metabolite removal [4, 11]. Although some of the units are portable and easy to use, it is recommended to consult with a certified professional before use, and ideally it should be performed by a certified professional for a young tennis player.

Summary

Tennis is an individual sport and requires an individual plan. For the young tennis player, an understanding of growth and development must be at the forefront of any periodization and planning process. It is a long process of development and requires patience, especially as a child is going through puberty. It is very important to remember that a child is not a miniature adult. Periodization will help to create an appropriate plan for a young tennis player based on individual needs. However, consistent reviews and adjustments are necessary. Recovery is a key component of the periodization plan. It is always important to remember that training does not improve an athlete without appropriate recovery. It is important to understand the benefits of different recovery methods and apply them at the appropriate time and in the appropriate amount. When coaches, parents, strength and conditioning coaches, and other support members for a young tennis player work together, they can develop and create a plan specific to the child and his or her overall development.

References

1. Baechle TR, Earle RW. Weight training step to success. 3rd ed. Champaign: Human Kinetics; 2006.
2. Baechel TR, Earle RW, Wathen D. Resistance training. In: Baechle TR, Earle RW, editors. Essential of strength training and conditioning. 3rd ed. Champaign: Human Kinetics; 2008. p. 381–412.
3. Bayli I, Hamilton AE. Long-term athlete development, trainability and physical preparation of tennis players. In: Reid M, Quinn A, Crespo M, editors. Strength and conditioning for tennis. London: ITF; 2003. p. 49–57.
4. Calder A. Coaching perspective of tennis recovery. In: Kovacs MS, Ellenbecker TS, Kibler WB, editors. Tennis recovery: a comprehensive review of the research. White Plains: United States Tennis Association Incorporated; 2010. p. 1–64.
5. Dieffenbach K. Physiological perspective of recovery in tennis. In: Kovacs MS, Ellenbecker TS, Kibler WB, editors. Tennis recovery: a comprehensive review of the research. White Plains: United States Tennis Association Incorporated; 2010. p. 210–82.
6. Faigenbaum A, Kraemer W, Blimkie CJR, Jeffereys I, Micheli LJ, Nitka M, Rowland TW. Youth resistance training: updated position statement paper the national strength and conditioning association. J Strength Cond Res. 2009;23(5):S60–79.
7. Ford P, Croix MDT, Llyoyd R, Meyers R, Moosavi M, Oliver J, Till K, Williams C. The long-term athletic development model: physiological evidence and application. J Sports Sci. 2011;29(4):389–402.
8. Gonzalez R, Ochoa C. Working with special populations – children, female, veterans and wheelchair players. Part I: children – physical activity and performance. In: Reid M, Quinn A, Crespo M, editors. Strength and conditioning for tennis. London: ITF; 2003. p. 187–92.
9. Hainline B. Positioning youth tennis for success. White Plains: United States Tennis Association Incorporated; 2013.
10. Hecimovich M. Sport specialization in youth: a literature review. J Am Chiropr Assoc. 2004;41(4):32–41.
11. ITPA. Certified tennis performance specialist (CTPS) workbook and study guide. ITPA. Atlanta: International Tennis Performance Association; 2012.
12. Jayanthi N, Dechert A, Durazo R, Dugas L, Luke A. Training and sports specialization risks in junior elite tennis players. J Med Sci Tennis. 2011;16(1):14–20.
13. Jayanthi N, Feller E, Smith A. Junior competitive tennis: ideal tournament and training recommendations. J Med Sci Tennis. 2013;18(2):30–5.
14. Jayanthi N, Pinkham C, Dugas L, Patrick B, LaBella C. Sport specialization in young athletes: evidence-based recommendations. Sport Health. 2012;5(3):251–7.
15. Kellmann M. Underrecovery and overtraining: different concept-similar impact? Olympic Coach. 2003;15(3):4–11.
16. Kovacs MS, Baker LB. Recovery interventions and strategies for improved tennis performance. Br J Sports Med. 2014;45:i18–21.
17. Kovacs MS, Ellenbecker TS, Kibler WB, Roetert EP, Lubbers P. Injury trends in american competitive junior tennis players. J Med Sci Tennis. 2014;19(1):19–24.
18. Kraemer WJ, Fleck SJ. Strength training for young athletes. 2nd ed. Champaign: Human Kinetics; 2005.

19. Lloyd RS, Oliver JL. The youth physical development model: a new approach to long-term athletic development. Strength Cond J. 2012;34(3):61–72.
20. Malina RM. Early sport specialization: roots, effectiveness, risks. Curr Sports Med Rep. 2010;9(6):364–71.
21. Ochi S, Campbell MJ. The progressive physical development of a high performance tennis player. Strength Cond J. 2009;31(4):59–68.
22. Otis CL, Crespo M, Flygare CT, Johnston PR, Kerber A, Loyd-Kolkin D, Loehr J, Martin K, Plum BM, Quinn A, Roetert P, Stroria KA, Terry PC. The Sony Ericsson WTA tour 10 year age eligibility and professional development review. Br J Sports Med. 2006;40:464–8.
23. Rowland TW. Children's exercise physiology. 2nd ed. Champaign: Human Kinetics; 2004.
24. Verstegen M. Developing strength. In: Reid M, Quinn A, Crespo M, editors. Strength and conditioning for tennis. London: ITF; 2003. p. 113–35.
25. Wathen D, Baechle TR, Earle RW. Periodization. In: Baechle TR, Earle RW, editors. Essentials of strength training and conditioning. 3rd ed. Champaign: Human Kinetics; 2008. p. 507–22.

Chapter 6
Acute Medical Problems in the Adolescent Tennis Player

Deena C. Casiero

Introduction

Tennis is one of the most popular individual sports in the world. It is a physically demanding sport that poses many challenges for adolescent players and requires peak physical fitness and mental readiness. It is commonly played outside in warm weather, and adolescent athletes are often expected to play multiple matches per day many of which can last several hours apiece. Therefore, in addition to the acute medical issues that can arise for any adolescent athlete (gastrointestinal, genitourinary, dermatologic, etc), the sport of tennis can expose players to specific demands that any health-care provider caring for these athletes should be familiar with.

Some of the most common acute medical problems that occur in adolescent tennis players are those involving fluid disorders. This can range from dehydration to cramping to acute heat illness. Education, fast recognition, and efficient management of these issues can be lifesaving in athletes with these conditions. Education and therefore prevention of fluid disorders and heat-related illness would have a huge impact on the morbidity and mortality of these conditions.

Congenital cardiovascular conditions such as hypertrophic cardiomyopathy and anomalous coronary arteries are a common cause of sudden cardiac death in athletes. These diagnoses are difficult to make, and they often do not manifest signs or symptoms until sudden cardiac death occurs. However, screening adolescent athletes for these conditions and restricting athletes from activity when the diagnosis is made can be lifesaving in many cases.

Concussions, or mild traumatic brain injuries, are not very common in the sport of tennis. However, a concussion can be sustained on the way to tennis practice or a

D.C. Casiero, MD
Primary Care Sports Medicine, ProHEALTH Care Associates,
2800 Marcus Avenue, Suite 102, Lake Success, NY 11042, USA
e-mail: Dcasiero@prohealthcare.com

© Springer International Publishing Switzerland 2016
A.C. Colvin, J.N. Gladstone (eds.), *The Young Tennis Player*: *Injury Prevention and Treatment*, Contemporary Pediatric and Adolescent Sports Medicine,
DOI 10.1007/978-3-319-27559-8_6

match from the result of a car accident or a accidently hitting one's head on a locker. It is important to learn how to diagnose and manage concussions in the tennis athlete to able to provide comprehensive care of the athlete.

Fluid Disorders and Heat-Related Illness

Junior competitive tennis is often played outdoors in warm climates, and even the fittest players will face challenges regarding the ability to appropriately replace water and electrolyte losses that occur during match play. In addition to their rigorous training schedules, tournament play poses the even more grueling challenge of multiple same-day matches [1]. When players are required to play more than one match per day with little time for rest and rehydration, there is an increased risk of heat-related illness from a phenomenon known as cumulative dehydration [2]. This occurs when the fluid and electrolyte losses from a match earlier in the day do not get fully replenished before the second match begins.

During both singles and doubles competitions being played in the heat, adolescent sweat losses have been reported as high as 1 L/h. Younger players are not always efficient at minimizing those fluid losses or replenishing them adequately during rest breaks [3]. The electrolytes lost through sweat must also be replaced in addition to water to maintain good hydration. Therefore, sports beverages containing sodium and chloride should be encouraged [3]. The combination of strong and constant exposure to the sun, high humidity levels, and degree of dehydration can lead to a variety of medical issues that vary in severity from exertional heat cramps to the potentially fatal exertional heat stroke [1].

Exertional Heat Cramps

Exertional heat cramps or exercise-associated muscle cramping (EAMC) is a common acute medical condition in adolescent tennis players. This type of muscle cramping can occur in fatigued muscles in the setting of electrolyte abnormalities, poor hydration, and unfavorable environmental conditions such as heat and humidity. Underlying metabolic disorders in the athlete must also be considered as a contributing cause [4].

Risk factors for EAMC includes a previous history of the disorder, exercise above and beyond the level at which the athlete has been training, and exercise in environmental conditions that puts the athlete at risk for electrolyte disorders and dehydration [5, 6]. Athletes with greater than average sweat rates, or athletes who are referred to as "salty sweaters," are also at an increased risk because of a larger total body sodium deficit [5].

Exercise-associated muscle cramping typically presents as generalized, bilateral cramping and often involve several large muscle groups at a time [5]. The athlete will often report a twitching sensation in the muscle during rest breaks, which may quickly progress to spasmodic contractions of the muscle if not treated promptly with rest and hydration [4–7]. Usually the cramping period will be followed by a period of relief once the activity has ceased and treatment has begun.

The first step in the treatment of EAMC is rest. Once the offending activity is stopped, passive stretching of the affected muscles should begin. Passive muscle stretching may take 20–30 min to allow full cessation of the fasciculations that occur in the affected muscles [4]. Cryotherapy is often applied to affected muscles to ease the discomfort associated with cramping until rehydration occurs [4, 5]. Oral fluid and electrolyte replacement is preferred over intravenous treatment in all athletes who are awake, alert, and able to tolerate oral fluids [4, 5]. Consuming 16–20 ounces of sport drink with an added half teaspoon of salt is usually adequate to treat EAMC [5].

As usual, prevention is always the best treatment for any acute medical condition. Adequate maintenance of fluid and electrolyte balance and achieving a peak level of fitness and conditioning should decrease the chance of an athlete suffering from EAMC. Routine consumption of a sport drink with 1150 mg of sodium per liter is typically well tolerated and helps to maintain hydration when playing in the heat [5]. Athletes prone to EAMC will need to pay special attention to their hydration status several days leading up to training and or competition, as the results of subsequent days of dehydration can be cumulative. Preparing the athlete to be at peak physical fitness for an upcoming event expected to occur in a warm and humid climate will help battle the muscle fatigue that can often play a role in EAMC [4]. Return to play may be considered once the muscle cramping has ceased and the athlete has been adequately rehydrated with both water and electrolytes [5].

Heat Exhaustion

Heat exhaustion can occur in adolescent tennis players who perform strenuous exercise in environmental conditions that include heat and humidity. It is typically defined as the inability to maintain cardiac output in the setting of moderate body temperatures [8]. The clinical manifestations of heat exhaustion include obvious difficulty with exercise, a moderate rise in core body temperature (101–104 °F), and no significant neurological symptoms. Other potential signs and symptoms of heat exhaustion are listed in Table 6.1.

Once an athlete begins to exhibit signs of heat exhaustion, it is imperative to remove the athlete from the warm environment and begin treatment right away in order to prevent the progression to more serious heat illness. The first step in treatment should be to move the athlete to a shaded or cooled area. Lay the athlete supine and elevate their legs to help direct the flow of blood towards the head [8]. Tennis players, unlike other athletes, do not normally wear excessive clothing or equipment when they play which is advantageous. However, if any excessive clothing is present, it should be removed. Core body temperature should only be taken using a

Table 6.1 Signs and symptoms of heat exhaustion	Obvious difficulty continuing to exercise
	Tachycardia
	Hypotension
	Dehydration or electrolyte imbalances
	Poor coordination
	Lightheadedness or syncope
	Profuse sweating
	Pallor
	Headache
	Abdominal cramps
	Nausea, vomiting, diarrhea
	Persistent muscle cramping

rectal thermometer. Alternative methods of obtaining core body temperature (e.g., oral, tympanic, axillary, etc) are not valid and may lead to an underestimate of the need for more intense cooling [9]. Cool the patient until his or her rectal temperature is approximately 101 °F.

The method chosen to cool the athlete is less important in heat exhaustion than in the more severe exertional heat stroke which will be discussed later in this chapter. Any technique used to cool an athlete with heat exhaustion is likely to be effective. This includes ice bags, cold shower, or cold-water immersion tubs. As long as the athlete is awake and alert, he or she should be rehydrated orally with a chilled sports drink while the cooling process continues.

Adolescent athletes that respond to the above treatments and show complete resolution of their symptoms within 1–2 h do not need further observation and may be sent home with a responsible adult. Athletes who do not respond to treatment or who decompensate should be cooled more vigorously before transportation to the hospital is initialized [9].

Prevention of heat exhaustion is most successful when the athletes are prepared for competition or training by being at peak physical fitness, properly hydrated, and educated regarding the best ways to take advantage of shade and cooling techniques before the symptoms begin.

Exertional Heat Stroke

Exertional heat stroke is defined as a multisystem illness that involves central nervous system dysfunction and end-organ damage, such as acute kidney injury, in the setting of core body temperatures above 104 °F [8, 10]. If heat exhaustion is not recognized and treated promptly, exertional heat stroke may result if the athlete continues to exercise in extreme weather conditions. The central nervous system dysfunction that occurs in heat stroke can present in a variety of ways including headache, confusion, emotional instability, disorientation, altered consciousness,

Table 6.2 Signs and symptoms of exertional heat stroke

Tachycardia
Hypotension
Tachypnea
Dizziness
Nausea, vomiting, diarrhea
Weakness
Profuse sweating
Headache
Irrational behavior
Disorientation
Irritability
Confusion
Altered consciousness
Coma
Seizure

and even seizure. A summary of the symptoms commonly found in exertional heat stroke can be found in Table 6.2.

Exertional heat stroke is a life-threatening illness, and despite progress with educating athletes, coaches, parents, and health-care providers, deaths from heat-related illness still appear to be rising [11]. Between the years 2005 and 2009, the US Centers for Disease Control reported an average of 9237 cases of exertional heat illness per year, and the number of deaths associated with these cases was higher than any other 5-year period over the past 35 years [12].

The key to effective treatment of this life-threatening illness is fast recognition of the diagnosis and rapid adequate cooling. As with any acute medical illness, the initial assessment of the athlete begins with evaluating and securing the airway, breathing, and circulation. Measurements of the athlete's vital signs should include a rectal temperature. As previously mentioned, other methods of temperature measurement are not accurate and should be avoided [9, 13]. If a rectal thermometer is not available and exertional heat stroke is thought to be the cause of the athlete's symptoms, cooling until shivering occurs (usually 10–15 min) is the suggested treatment [14].

If a rectal thermometer is available and the core body temperature is above 105 °F, in the setting of altered mental status, this is consistent with a diagnosis of exertional heat stroke. Rapid cooling must begin immediately. This is the most effective strategy for minimizing morbidity and mortality in an athlete with exertional heat stroke [14]. If appropriate medical staff and supplies are present on-site and no other medical emergencies other than exertional heat stroke are present, it is usually best to follow the "cool-first, transport-second" guideline [10].

There are few controlled studies available regarding the best method to cool an athlete suffering from exertional heat stroke, but several systemic reviews have concluded that ice water immersion may be the most effective method [15]. If immersion in an ice water bath is not feasible, other methods such as dousing the athlete with

Table 6.3 Key steps in cooling an athlete with exertional heat stroke

Activate EMS
If appropriate medical staff is on-site: cool-first, transport second
Remove all excess clothing
Immerse athlete in tub of cold water (35–60 °F)
Cover as much of the body as possible
Keep the athletes head and neck above water
Place a towel soaked in ice water over the head and neck while the body is being cooled
If an immersion tub is not available, initiate alternative method of cooling immediately (dousing, ice towels, etc)
Monitor vital signs every 10 min (rectal temperature, heart rate, respiratory rate, blood pressure)
Monitor mental status
Maintain patient safety at all times
Cease cooling when rectal temperature reaches 101°–102 °F
Transfer athlete to the hospital

cold water, application of cold wet towels, or ice bags have been described [15]. A summary of the key steps involved in cooling an athlete with exertional heat stroke can be found in Table 6.3. It is important to remember to maintain the safety of the athlete at all times during the cooling process. This means the athlete's head may need to be physically held out of the water while he or she is being immersed in the cold-water tub. Using a towel draped around the chest and under the axillae is an effective way to support the athlete during cooling.

In summary, a variety of heat-related illnesses could occur in adolescent tennis athletes especially if they are dehydrated or deconditioned. These illnesses range from benign exercise-associated muscle cramping to the potentially fatal exertional heat stroke. However, the best way to manage these acute medical illnesses is to prevent them by focusing on educating athletes, coaches, and parents. The number of heat-related illnesses that occur each year could be significantly reduced by continued efforts to ensure that our athletes are well conditioned, acclimatized to their environment, and properly hydrated going into training or competition.

Acute Cardiovascular Events

Sudden cardiac death in athletes is rare with an incidence reported to be between 1 per 50,000 and 1 per 300,000 athletes over a 15-year period [16]. The most common exercise-related cardiovascular events that occur in adolescent athletes are typically congenital and not diagnosed until after the event. A US registry of sudden cardiac death in 1435 young competitive athletes documented hypertrophic cardiomyopathy and anomalous coronary arteries as the two most commonly seen underlying congenital conditions contributing to 36 % and 17 % of cases respectively [17]. Although there are many acute cardiovascular conditions that may cause sudden

Table 6.4 Twelve major points of the pre-participation screening exam for high school and collegiate athletes

Personal history elements
1. Exertional chest pain
2. Unexplained syncope/near syncope
3. Excessive exertional and unexplained dyspnea/fatigue associated with exercise
4. Prior recognition of a heart murmur
5. Elevated systemic blood pressure
Family history elements:
6. Premature death in a relative under the age of 50 due to heart disease
7. Disability from heart disease in a close relative under the age of 50
8. Specific knowledge of cardiac conditions in family members (hypertrophic or dilated cardiomyopathy, long QT syndrome, arrhythmias)
Physical exam elements:
9. Heart murmur (supine, standing, valsalva)
10. Femoral pulses to exclude aortic coarctation
11. Physical stigmata of Marfan syndrome
12. Brachial blood pressure (sitting, both arms)

cardiac death in the adolescent tennis athlete, this chapter will focus on the two most common conditions.

Most adolescent athletes who have these underlying congenital abnormalities are largely asymptomatic and are unaware that they are at increased risk for sudden cardiac death. Hence, the pre-participation physical exam is important in the identification of an at-risk population. In 2007, the American Heart Association guidelines for pre-participation screening in adolescent athletes were updated with a focus on personal and family history of cardiac symptoms or conditions and a physical examination to evaluate for heart murmur [17]. Table 6.4 is a summary of all 12 key focal points of the pre-participation exam. Routine use of an EKG for screening purposes is not recommended [17].

Hypertrophic Cardiomyopathy

Hypertrophic cardiomyopathy (HCM) has been reported in as many as 1 in 350 to 1 in 625 people in the USA [18]. Most adolescent athletes with HCM are asymptomatic but occasionally may present with dyspnea on exertion, fatigue, atypical or anginal chest pain, palpitations, presyncope, or syncope (particularly during or immediately following exertion). These symptoms occur because of the underlying structural changes that occur in the heart including left ventricular outflow obstruction, diastolic dysfunction, and mitral regurgitation, and in severe cases, myocardial ischemia is a possibility.

The physical exam of an athlete with HCM can be completely normal or may reveal nonspecific abnormalities such as a fourth heart sound or a systolic murmur. The classic murmur that is described is usually only heard when significant left ventricular outflow tract obstruction is present. This results in a harsh crescendo-decrescendo systolic murmur, is heard best at the apex and lower left sternal border, and begins slightly after S1. The murmur may radiate to the axilla and base but usually does not radiate into the neck [19].

In order to further evaluate a murmur heard on pre-participation physical exam screening, the athlete may be asked to perform a set of maneuvers that affect the degree of outflow tract obstruction. If present, these maneuvers should cause a change in intensity of the outflow tract crescendo-decrescendo murmur. Asking the athlete to perform a Valsalva maneuver should increase the intensity of the murmur by enhancing the obstruction, while asking them to perform a handgrip maneuver should decrease the intensity due to attenuation of the obstruction [19].

During the screening process, a common challenge becomes distinguishing between left ventricular hypertrophy secondary to HCM and the commonly seen increase in left ventricular wall thickness, cavity size, and mass seen in well-trained athletes. This is often referred to as "athletic heart syndrome." Further cardiovascular testing such as a 12-lead electrocardiogram, echocardiogram, and occasionally functional exercise testing is often needed to distinguish these two entities.

Though the data is limited, activity is often restricted in athletes diagnosed with HCM [20]. The recommendations to restrict all but extremely low-intensity activity apply to athletes of all ages and do not differ by sex. Whether or not the athlete has any symptoms, LV outflow obstruction, or prior treatment with drugs, or major interventions including implantation of a pacemaker, or implantable cardioverter-defibrillator, does not change the recommendations.

Congenital Coronary Artery Abnormalities

Anomalous coronary arteries have been reported in 12–33 % of young athletes who have suffered sudden cardiac death [21–23]. There are many different types of anomalous coronary arteries, but the two most common are the origin of the left main coronary artery from the right sinus of Valsalva and the origin of the right coronary artery from the left coronary sinus [24].

Those anomalies considered to be high risk are those in which the anomalous coronary artery makes an acute bend and courses between the pulmonary artery and aorta [25]. During exercise, the aorta and pulmonary trunk expand, further exaggerating the sharp angle that occurs at the aberrant origin of the anomalous artery which may cause ischemia and cardiac cell death.

Physical examination and diagnostic studies are usually unrevealing in the absence of symptoms of prolonged ischemia or frank myocardial infarction.

Unfortunately, sudden cardiac death is usually the first clinical symptom in athletes with congenital coronary anomalies. However, clinical presentation may include anginal chest pain, syncope, or presyncope, especially with exercise. In a study looking at autopsy results on 27 patients with an anomalous coronary artery, more than half (55 %) exhibited no clinical manifestations during life or with testing. In the remaining 12 patients, premonitory symptoms, such as syncope and chest pain, occurred only shortly before death despite all cardiovascular testing being negative at the time of symptoms [26].

When anomalous origin of a coronary artery is suspected, noninvasive imaging using magnetic resonance coronary angiography or coronary angiography by computed tomography can be used to make the diagnosis. Coronary angiography had been the gold standard in the past and is still used when noninvasive testing is not diagnostic [27].

Recommendations published by the 2005 36th Bethesda Conference state that any athlete with uncorrected anomalous coronary artery origin be excluded from competitive sports despite the presence or absence of symptoms [27]. Surgical correction with bypass grafting is considered appropriate management in some cases. Three months after surgical correction, if the athlete shows no signs of infarction, ischemia, arrhythmia, or left ventricular dysfunction during maximal exercise testing, he or she may be evaluated on a case-by-case basis for return to play [27].

Screening adolescent athletes for underlying cardiac abnormalities during the pre-participation physical is extremely important. Identifying those athletes at greatest risk and removing them from competition could be potentially lifesaving. Some conditions, however, despite appropriate screening, will go unnoticed. Unfortunately, the first clinical symptom of these conditions may be sudden cardiac death. Having a well-rehearsed emergency action plan for all practices and competitive events will help minimize fatalities in some of these cases. Coaches and medical personnel should be well trained in cardiopulmonary resuscitation and be familiar with how to operate an automatic electronic defibrillator. Once a fatal arrhythmia occurs, despite its underlying cause, these skills will provide the best chance at successful resuscitation of the athlete.

Sports-Related Concussion

Though sport-related concussion accounts for 13–15 % of all injuries sustained by high school athletes, the incidence in the sport of tennis is much lower [28]. Tennis is an individual noncontact sport that does not typically put the athlete at risk for head injury during play. However, tennis athletes can become concussed in a variety of ways off court that can affect their performance and overall health if not diagnosed and addressed properly.

Definition of Concussion

Based on the consensus statement from the 4th International Conference on Concussion in Sport, the definition of a concussion is brain injury in which a complex pathophysiological process affecting the brain was induced by biomechanical forces [29]. Concussions can be caused either by a direct blow to the head, face, neck, or elsewhere on the body which may produce a reactive force that is then transmitted to the head. Concussion can result in the rapid onset of short-lived impairment of neurological function that resolves spontaneously or symptoms may evolve over a number of minutes to hours. Typically, the acute clinical symptoms largely reflect a functional disturbance rather than a structural injury, and normally no abnormality is seen on imaging of the brain. The symptoms of a concussion are longer graded and may or may not involve loss of consciousness. The clinical and cognitive symptoms typically resolve sequentially, but in certain athletes, the time course can be prolonged [29].

Grading

In the past, concussions were graded by severity as mild (grade 1), moderate (grade 2), and severe (grade 3) based on the presence and duration of loss of consciousness. Recent literature suggests that clinical course and long-term cognitive impairment is not associated with loss of consciousness; therefore, grading of concussions has fallen out of favor [29, 30].

Pathophysiology

The pathophysiology of concussion is still not entirely understood. Some research shows that for days to weeks after a concussion, there is a decrease in cerebral blood flow. Since glucose is delivered to the brain via the blood stream, the increased demand for glucose and its end product, ATP, go unfulfilled. This mismatch in supply and demand is thought to result in the cognitive dysfunction and symptoms of a concussion [31].

Evaluation

Once a concussion is suspected, the player should be removed from play immediately, and a sideline or training room evaluation should be performed by a trained member of the health-care team. A summary of the most common signs and symptoms of a concussion can be found in Table 6.5.

Table 6.5 Common signs and symptoms of concussion	Headache
	Confusion and disorientation
	Difficulty with memory (short or long term)
	Blank stare or "dazed" appearance
	Inattentiveness
	Slow or incoherent speech
	Dizziness
	Gait abnormalities and imbalance (stumbling, falling)
	Nausea
	Vomiting
	Emotional lability (inappropriate laughing or crying)

Physical Exam

Physical examination of an athlete with a suspected concussion should always begin with observation. Note his or her speech pattern, behavior, affect, and mood as these may all be altered in the setting of acute head trauma. A detailed neurologic exam with close attention to the cranial nerves should be performed to evaluate for any signs of intracranial bleeding. Although this is a rare complication of concussion, it must not be overlooked. Strength testing of the upper and lower extremities as well as evaluation of the vestibular and occulomotor systems should be included [32].

Cognitive evaluation should include questions addressing orientation (to person, place, and time), memory evaluation (both short and long term), and concentration. An example of a commonly used question to assess memory is asking the athlete to repeat a set of five words in any order he or she can remember them. This is repeated three times with the same five words each time. Later in the evaluation, the athlete is asked once again to repeat back the same five words. This tests both long-term and short-term memory. To test concentration, the athlete can be asked to recite the months of the year backwards starting with December. This task challenges the athlete to both concentrate and remain attentive.

Cognitive evaluation can also be performed using a tool such as the Sport Concussion Assessment Tool 3 (SCAT3). This tool has not been validated in prospective trials but was endorsed in the 2012 Consensus Statement on Concussion in Sport and is widely used for sideline evaluation [33]. It provides a well-organized and detailed guide to clinical assessment and includes: a review of indications for emergency referral, Glasgow Coma Scale, symptom assessment, and physical and cognitive assessment. It is a comprehensive tool that helps to perform an organized concussion evaluation.

Balance testing is a key component to the sideline evaluation. The Balance Error Scoring System (BESS) has been validated and has proven to be reliable in athletes with more severe balance disturbances. The test is easy to perform and only takes a few minutes to complete. The athlete is asked to close his or her eyes and do the following on both soft and firm surfaces for 20 s with the hands placed on the hips: single-leg stance, double-leg stance, and tandem stance. An error is recorded each time the athlete opens their eyes, lifts their hands off of their iliac crests, stumbles, moves into greater than 30° of hip flexion or abduction, lifts their heel or forefoot, or remains out of position for more than 5 s [34]. Because of the individual variation among athletes on tests, baseline testing is useful to measure trends in performance.

Baseline and Neuropsychological Testing

Baseline neuropsychological testing refers to testing that is performed on all athletes prior to injury and is used as a comparison if the athlete develops a concussion at a later date. These tests examine skills such as memory, concentration, balance, and reaction time. Since cognitive recovery can lag behind physical recovery, many physicians use neuropsychological tests as a tool to monitor an athlete's progress. These tests are not used as an absolute diagnostic tool. Instead, they are meant to be used in conjunction with the clinical history and physical exam and to aid in decision making for return to play [35].

Diagnosis

Before a diagnosis of concussion is made, a history of direct or indirect trauma in conjunction with the onset of signs and symptoms of a concussion should be taken into account. Also, standardized assessments of symptoms, balance, and neurocognitive function should point towards a diagnosis of concussion while other intracranial injuries (i.e., intracranial bleeding) have been excluded with or without the use of neuroimaging.

Management

Once the diagnosis of a concussion is made, it is imperative that it be managed appropriately to provide the best chance of a full and uncomplicated recovery. The management of concussions in the adolescent athlete is based on observational studies, clinical experience, and consensus guidelines [28, 29, 36]. The first step in management once the athlete has been cleared of any other serious injury, such as a cervical spine injury, is to make sure the athlete does not return to play until full recovery has occurred. Athletes should never be allowed to return to play on the day of their injury even if they report complete symptom resolution. The athlete must first be evaluated by a health-care professional with experience managing concussion and may need to complete a progressive return to play protocol prior to returning to sport. Physical and cognitive rest, with a slow and progressive return to play, are the primary interventions for concussion.

Typically, no exercise is permitted while the athlete continues to report symptoms of concussion. The duration of symptoms is very individualized and can vary drastically in different athletes but usually lasts between 7 and 14 days [36]. Normal activities of daily living are permitted during this stage. Normal sleep is recommended, while the athlete is symptomatic and he or she is encouraged to get as much rest as possible. Cognitive rest is typically recommended as well, especially in adolescent athletes with concussion [37]. However, one must consider the consequences of missing significant time away from school, and the amount of time the athlete is held out can usually be determined on an individual basis.

Once the athlete no longer reports any signs or symptoms of concussion and has returned to baseline on the concussion assessment tools, he or she should be reevaluated by a physician. Once the physician documents that the athlete and the appropriate testing has returned to baseline, a return to play protocol can be initiated [29, 38]. Return to play protocols are usually sport specific and begin with an aerobic challenge such as bike riding. If asymptomatic upon the completion of this task, the next day he or she may perform a more challenging task such as running or sprinting. If over the next 24 h, the athlete remains asymptomatic, he or she should be allowed to perform some sports specific drills such as practicing strokes or serves. Eventually he will be placed into practice-like situations that will require all the skills and aerobic capacity needed to return to competitive tennis. Once he is able to practice at 100 % of his capacity without symptoms, he should be seen by a physician for a final evaluation and cleared to return to play without restriction at that time. A typical return to play protocol may take anywhere from 5 to 7 days to complete.

Concussions are serious injuries that plague athletes of all sports. Adolescent tennis players are not at increased risk for concussion given the nature of their sport. However, all health-care providers caring for adolescent tennis players should be able to recognize and manage a player with a concussion in order to provide complete care of the young athlete. Education of the athletes, coaches and medical community continues to be the single most important aspect of concussion management.

References

1. Bergeron MF. Hydration and thermal strain during tennis in the heat. Br J Sports Med. 2014;48:i12–7.
2. Bergeron MF, McLeod KS, Coyle JF. Core body temperature during competition in the heat: national boy's 14's junior tennis championships. Br J Sports Med. 2007;41:779–83.
3. Bergeron MF, Waller JL, Marinik EL. Voluntary fluid intake and core temperature responses in adolescent tennis players: sports beverage versus water. Br J Sports Med. 2006;40:406–10.
4. Schwellnus MP, Drew N, Collins M. Muscle cramping in athletes—risk factors, clinical assessment, and management. Clin Sports Med. 2008;27:183–94.
5. Bergeron MF. Exertional heat cramps: recovery and return to play. J Sport Rehabil. 2007;16:190–6.
6. Bergeron MF. Heat cramps: fluid and electrolyte challenges during tennis in the heat. J Sci Med Sport. 2003;6(1):19–27.

7. American College of Sports Medicine, Armstrong LE, Casa DJ, Millard-Stafford M, Moran DS, Pyne SW, et al. American College of Sports Medicine position stand. Exertional heat illness during training and competition. Med Sci Sports Exerc. 2007;39:556–72.
8. Winkenwerder W, Sawka M. Disorders due to heat and cold. In: Goldman L, editor. Cecil medicine. Philadelphia: Saunders Elsevier; 2008. p. 668–70.
9. Casa DJ, Becker SM, Ganio MS, Brown CM, Yeargin SW, Roti MW, et al. Validity of devices that assess body temperature during outdoor exercise in the heat. J Athl Train. 2007;42(3):333–42.
10. Bouchama A, Knochel JP. Heat stroke. N Engl J Med. 2002;346(25):1978–88.
11. Mueller FO, Cantu RC. Catastrophic sports injury research: 26th annual report fall 1982-spring 2008. Chapel Hill: University of North Carolina; 2008. http://www.unc.Edu/depts./nccsi/Allsport.pdf. Accessed on 13 Aug 2014.
12. Centers for Disease Control and Prevention (CDC). Heat illness among high school athletes-United States, 2005-2009. MMWR Morb Mortal Wkly Rep. 2010;59:1009.
13. Mazerolle SM, Ganio MS, Casa DJ, Vingren J, Klau J. Is oral temperature an accurate measurement of deep body temperature? A systematic review. J Athl Train. 2011;46(5):566–73.
14. Casa DJ, Kenny GP, Taylor NA. Immersion treatment for exertional hyperthermia: cold or temperate water? Med Sci Sports Exerc. 2010;42:1246–52.
15. Smith JE. Cooling methods used in the treatment of exertional heat illness. Br J Sports Med. 2005;39:503–7.
16. Van Camp SP, Bloor CM, Mueller FO, Cantu RC, Olson HG. Nontraumatic sports death in high school and college athletes. Med Sci Sports Exerc. 1995;27(5):641–7.
17. Maron BJ, Thompson PD, Ackerman MJ, Balady G, Berger S, Cohen D. Recommendations and considerations related to preparticipation screening for cardiovascular abnormalities in competitive athletes: 2007 update: a scientific statement from the American Heart Association council on nutrition, physical activity and metabolism: endorsed by the American College of Cardiology Foundation. Circulation. 2007;115:1643–55.
18. Maron BJ, Gardin JM, Flack JM, Gidding SS. Prevalence of hypertrophic cardiomyopathy in a general population of young adults. Circulation. 1995;92(4):785.
19. Lim V, Rao Kokkirala A, Thompson PD. Cardiovascular system. In: Mckeag DB, Moeller JL, editors. ACSM's primary care sports medicine. Philadelphia: Lippincott Williams & Wilkins; 2007. p. 189.
20. Maron BJ, Ackerman MJ, Nishimura RA, Pyeritz RE, Towbin JA, Udelson JE. Task Force 4: HCM and other cardiomyopathies, mitral valve prolapse, myocarditis, and marfan's syndrome. J Am Coll Cardiol. 2005;45(8):1340–5.
21. Eckart RE, Scoville SL, Campell CL, Shry EA, Stajduhar KC, Potter RN, et al. Sudden death in young adults: a 25-year review of autopsies in military recruits. Ann Intern Med. 2004;141:829–34.
22. Corrado D, Basso C, Schiavon M, Thiene G. Screening for hypertrophic cardiomyopathy in young athletes. N Engl J Med. 1998;339(6):364–9.
23. Maron BJ, Carney KP, Lever HM, Lewis JF, Barac I, Casey SA, et al. Relationship of race to sudden cardiac death in competitive athletes with hypertrophic cardiomyopathy. J Am Coll Cardiol. 2003;41(6):974–80.
24. Taylor JA, Rogan KM, Virmani R. Sudden cardiac death associated with isolated congenital coronary artery anomalies. J Am Coll Cardiol. 2002;20(3):640–7.
25. Taylor JA, Byers JP, Cheitlin MD, Virmani R. Anomalous right or left coronary from the contralateral coronary sinus: "high-risk" abnormalities in the initial coronary artery course and heterogeneous clinical outcomes. Am Heart J. 2007;133:428–35.
26. Basso C, Maron BJ, Corrado D, Thiene G. Clinical profile of congenital coronary artery anomalies with origin from the wrong aortic sinus leading to sudden cardiac death in young competitive athletes. J Am Coll Cardiol. 2000;35(6):1493–501.
27. Graham TP, Driscoll DJ, Gersony WM, Newburger JW, Rocchini A, Towbin JA. J Am Coll Cardiol. 2005;45(8):1326–33.

28. Meehan WP, d'Hemecourt P, Collins CL, Comstock RD. Assessment and management of sports related concussion in United States high schools. Am J Sports Med. 2011;39:2304–10.
29. McCrory P, Meeuwisse W, Aubry M, Cantu B, Dvorak J, Echemendia RJ, et al. Consensus statement on concussion in sport-the 4th international conference on concussion in sport held in Zurich, November 2012. Clin J Sport Med. 2013;23(2):89–117.
30. Gomez JE, Hergenroeder AC. New guidelines for management of concussion in sport: special concern for youth. J Adolesc Health. 2013;53(3):311–3.
31. Yuan XQ, Prough DS, Smith TL, Dewitt DS. The effects of traumatic brain injury on regional cerebral blood flow in rats. J Neurotrauma. 1988;5(4):289–301.
32. Alsalaheen BA, Mucha A, Morris LO, Whitney SL, Furman JM, Camiolo-Reddy CE, et al. Vestibular rehabilitation for dizziness and balance disorders after concussion. J Neurol Phys Ther. 2010;34(2):87–93.
33. Guskiewicz KM, Register-Mihalik J, McCrory P, McCrea M, Johnston K, Makdissi M, et al. Evidence-based approach to revising the SCAT2: introducing the SCAT3. Br J Sports Med. 2013;47(5):289–93.
34. Bell DR, Guskiewicz KM, Clark MA, Padua DA. Systematic review of the balance error scoring system. Sports Health. 2011;3(3):287–95.
35. Van Kampen DA, Lovell MR, Pardini JE, Collins MW, Fu FH. The "value added" of neurocognitive testing after sports concussion. Am J Sports Med. 2006;34(10):1630–5.
36. Meehan WP, d'Hemecourt P, Comstock RD. High school concussions in the 2008-2009 academic year: mechanism, symptoms, and management. Am J Sports Med. 2010;38:2405–9.
37. Halstead ME, McAvoy K, Devore CD, Carl R, Lee M, Logan K, et al. Returning to learning following a concussion. Pediatrics. 2013;132:948–57.
38. Halstead ME, Walter KD. The council on sports medicine and fitness. Sport-related concussion in children and adolescents. Pediatrics. 2010;126:597–615.

Chapter 7
Spine Injuries in Tennis Players

Steven Mcanany, Diana Patterson, and Andrew C. Hecht

Introduction

Tennis is a sport played across the globe and with ever-increasing popularity. Elite adolescent tennis players who want to reach the professional ranks spend extensive hours performing strenuous and intense training, particularly during developmental stages and their pre-pubertal growth spurt. This, as well as the drive for ever-increasing racquet velocities, leads to higher demand on the lumbar spine [1].

Anatomy and Biomechanics

The spine is made up of 33 single vertebrae (though the coccygeal vertebrae are fused early in life). During motion, however, the vertebrae move together with its adjacent structures. In flexion and extension, each vertebra performs sagittal plane rotation and translation in relation to its next lower vertebrae [2]. In normal motion, the "instantaneous axis of rotation," the arc of the center of movement as a vertebra moves from point to point, is within the posterior part of the disc [3]. The spine acts as a kinetic chain in which motion at one point influences, and is influenced by,

S. Mcanany, MD
Department of Orthopaedic Surgery, Mount Sinai Medical Center, New York, USA

D. Patterson, MD
Resident Orthopaedic Surgery, Mount Sinai Medical Center, New York, USA

A.C. Hecht, MD (✉)
Department of Spine Surgery, Mount Sinai Health System, New York, USA

Mount Sinai Spine Center, New York, USA
e-mail: andrew.hecht@mountsinai.org

© Springer International Publishing Switzerland 2016
A.C. Colvin, J.N. Gladstone (eds.), *The Young Tennis Player: Injury Prevention and Treatment*, Contemporary Pediatric and Adolescent Sports Medicine,
DOI 10.1007/978-3-319-27559-8_7

121

movement at others along the line. The predominant movements of the spine are flexion, extension, lateral flexion, and rotation. These relationships are not uniform across all subjects, as there are inherent differences between men and women, the elderly and the young [4].

Biomechanical studies have shown that the movement of a vertebra follows a set pattern, described as a coupled motion, that is defined by the bony relationships and from attachments and actions of the peripheral elastic ligaments and muscles. The support mechanisms of the spine have been divided into three categories: passive, active, and neurological [5]. The spinal column, which includes the bony structures, joints, and ligamentous structures, provides passive, or intrinsic, stability, which is most critical at the end of range of motion. The paraspinal musculature, which supplies an active, dynamic stability, changes the stiffness of the spine in response to the bodies' needs. The neural system coordinates the muscular response to extern and internal forces. The interaction between these global and local systems provides dynamic stabilization. The local muscles, which include the deep back muscles and deep portions of muscles that insert on to the vertebrae, influence the rigidity and posture of the spinal segments. The global muscles, the larger superficial muscles that do not attach directly to vertebrae, generate torque, influence posture, balance loads applied to the trunk, and are critical in transferring loads from thorax to the pelvis [6]. Studies are undecided as to whether strength deficits of the back muscles are related or causal of low back pain. A study by Biering-Sorensen [7] found that deficits in back strength did not predict the appearance of back pain over 1 year, but Luoto et al. [8] showed that poor static basic endurance is related to onset of back pain. More recently, McGill et al. [9] revealed that low back pain is associated with reduced endurance of back extensors versus that of back flexors. In a study of 82 amateur tennis players with and without low back pain, Renkawitz et al. [10] found a significant association between neuromuscular imbalance of the erector spinae and the occurrence of low back pain, while no significant imbalance was found in the subjects without low back pain. After the subjects completed a back exercise program, the number of subjects with low back pain decreased proportionally with the occurrence of neuromuscular imbalance; those subjects who till reported low back pain also retained evidence of neuromuscular imbalance.

Tennis-Related Spine Injuries

Tennis is an acyclic and one-sided sport, requiring fast movements of the trunk in flexion and extension in both the sagittal and coronal planes, as well as rotational movements around the long axis [1]. Sports with such an emphasis on forward bending and extension are associated with alterations in changes in the spinal curves of sagittal plane and a resultant greater risk of injury to the spine [11]. A clinical study by Muyor et al. [1] of 40 adolescent tennis players measured the spinal curvatures and pelvic tilt in a relaxed staining posture and supine. It showed that there was no abnormal thoracic hyperkyphosis or associated lumbar hypo-/hyperlordosis in the young tennis athlete. There was, however, a greater thoracic kyphosis, lower lumbar lordosis, and lower pelvic tilt in the female subjects.

In tennis, the power to hit the ball with great force is created in the lower extremity and transferred through the trunk into the arm. Any missing or weakened link along this chain can result in reduction in force generation and an increase in injury risk. Additionally, tennis is an inherently repetitive sport, thereby also setting up players for overuse injuries. Rotational movement is essential, but repetitive aggressive rotation can also cause microtrauma and lead to instability without sufficient dynamic stabilization [12]. As a result, load transmission is shifted from the facet joints to the intervertebral discs and ligaments [13]. A kinematic study by Kawasaki et al. found that the one-handed backhand had significantly smaller extension moment before ball impact and smaller lateral bending and axial rotation moments after impact. Therefore, in the one-handed backhand, the shoulder and elbow share the rotational motion of stroke and reduce impact on the spine in comparison the two-handed backhand [14]. However, studies have not identified a correlation between handedness and side of injury, and there are no in vivo studies of injuries to the spine or trunk muscles in players who use one- or two-handed backhand. Other studies have shown that the serve, often the most frequently performed strokes, loads the lumbar spine the most, with lateral flexion forces that are approximately eight times greater than those encountered during running [15]. In particular, the topspin "kick serve" assigns the highest forces to the lumbar spine [16].

Injury Epidemiology

The majority of injuries occurring in tennis are muscle sprains and ligament strains in the lower extremity and trunk due to acute trauma or overuse. The back, trunk, and hips are critically important to the tennis athletes, as they are a center of rotation and transmit forces generated in the legs to the shoulder and arms to hit the ball with power and top spin. In a 2-year study of 12–18-year-old members of a tennis club, injury incidence was 1.7/1000 h of playing time and 0.6/1000 h of playing time for boys and girls, respectively. Low back pain, ankle sprains, and knee injuries were the most commonly reported injuries. Sixty five percent of these were new injuries, mostly at the knee, while the majority of the remaining recurrent injuries were in the lumbar spine [17]. The lumbar spine represents the third most common site of musculoskeletal injury in tennis players after lower and upper extremity injuries [18, 19]. Historically, low back pain has been reported in up to one-third of professional tennis players [20]. In more recent studies, reported incidence rates for low back pain range from 31 to 50 % [21].

Cervical and Thoracic Spine

There is very little data regarding injuries to the cervical and thoracic spine in tennis. Neck sprain and strains are possible considering the rotational nature of the sport, but are rare. Additionally, in the young patient, the majority of cervical spine injuries associated with sports are due to traumatic injuries, especially football or water sports involving headfirst diving. Thoracic spine injuries are rare overall, except in high-speed trauma. The ribs stabilize the thoracic spine and generally prevent the injuries that occur in the lumbar spine [22]. These are very unusual injuries in tennis players and are usually not part of the spectrum of injuries due to the non-contact nature of this sport.

Lumbar and Lumbosacral Spine

Injuries of the lumbar and lumbosacral spine are more common due to the repetitive nature of the tennis stroke. While there are reports of more acute traumatic injuries, such as fractures to facets and parts of the vertebral bodies, most tennis-related injuries are subacute or chronic in nature. Muscle strains and sprains of the abdominal and superficial back and paraspinal muscles are common and lead to a varying time away from play. More serious injuries include damage to the facet joints, disc herniations and degeneration, and spondylolysis or spondylolisthesis.

Radiographic Findings

Investigators have studied imaging studies of tennis athletes with and without symptoms and most pathology is localized to the lumbar spine. Studying the asymptomatic tennis athlete aids in the understanding of causal mechanisms and the formulation of injury prevention or rehabilitation protocols. There have been several published studies following imaging of asymptomatic young and adolescent tennis athletes. In a recent MRI study of 98 asymptomatic elite junior tennis players, only four players were without any lumbar spine pathology [23]. Facet joint arthropathy was found in 88 individuals. Synovial cysts were seen in 22 patients, all related to facet joint degeneration. There was abnormality of the pars interarticularis in 41 vertebrae, all but 3 occurring at the L5 level, with 11 being bilateral. Spondylolisthesis was seen in 5 of 98 patients, though all were grade 1. Lastly, 61 of the 98 players had MRI evidence of disc degeneration confined to at least 1 level with most at L5–S1. There were 36 disc herniations, 5 focal and the rest broad-based, and 7 subjects with nerve root impingement, all of those at L5–S1. Overall, the prevalence of these pathologies was lower in female subjects than the males and lower in the under 16-year-olds in comparison with those over 20 years of age. These MRI reports may demonstrate the early damage that repetitive microtrauma can cause. The overall prevalence of facet joint arthropathy is much higher than what is seen in studies involving an aged-matched population. Most likely, this is due to the twisting of intervertebral discs and repetitive facet joint loading that occurs with the serving motion, top spin shots, and double-handed backhands. This is also likely to be the case with the abnormalities of the pars interarticularis. An earlier study by Lundin et al. which compared MRIs of young athletes with a control group of non-athletes revealed that the athletes had significantly more radiological abnormalities but did not report a higher frequency of back pain than the non-athletes [24].

Spondylolysis and Spondylolisthesis

Spondylolysis is an anatomic defect in the pars interarticularis of the vertebral arch without displacement of the vertebral body. Upright ambulation is theorized to be a contributing factor. It is estimated to occur naturally in approximately 6 % of the population, increasing in prevalence from birth to approximately age 22. Physical activities that accentuate the natural lumbar lordosis through required hyperextension and rotational loads are thought to be a cause of pars defects, spondylolysis, and, potentially, spondylolisthesis [25]. A "stress reaction" refers to the incomplete bone disruption and sclerosis one might see on CT or the intraosseous edema on MRI, at the pars, lamina, or pedicle. A spondylolytic, or isthmic, defect is when it contains a radiolucent gap with sclerosis of the edges. Though there are five types of spondylolysthesis in the commonly used Wiltse-Newman classification, only types I and II are commonly applied to children (Table 7.1). Only type II, the isthmic type, is defined as resulting from a defect in the pars interarticularis, commonly occurring in young athletes. It is subdivided into type IIA, B, and C; type IIA is from a fatigue failure of the pars secondary to repetitive loading and can be diagnosed by a completely radiolucent defect; type IIB is caused by an elongated pars that occurs due to repeated micro fractures that heal; type IIC is an acute pars injury [26].

In addition to tennis, these injuries are commonly reported in gymnastics, diving, and football. With immobilization and cessation from activities, stress injuries may heal. However, when the defect is left untreated, healing is less predictable. The most commonly used radiographic classification to quantify severity of slippage was proposed by Meyerding in 1932 (Table 7.2). It is best calculated on a lateral radiograph. The degree of slippage is the percentage of distance that the anteriorly translated superior vertebral body has moved on the inferior vertebral body. Many patients also present with a low-grade spondylolisthetic slip, but only a small percentage continue to progress with age. The adolescent tennis athlete is most likely to present with low back pain, hamstring tightness, or pain radiating to the posterior thigh; it is also a diagnosis that should be considered in the athletic patient who reports repeated hamstring strains or inability to stretch fully or to rotate to one side over the other. Radicular symptoms or any incontinence of bowel or bladder is rare as the compression usually

Table 7.1 Wiltse-Newman classification of spondylolisthesis

Type		
I	Dysplastic	A: Facet with axial orientation
		B: Facet with sagittal orientation
II	Isthmic	A: Lytic
		B: Pars elongation
		C: Pars fracture
III	Degenerative	
IV	Traumatic	
V	Pathological	
VI	Postsurgical	

Table 7.2 Meyerding classification for spondylolisthesis

Grade	Percentage of slippage
Grade 0[a]	0 (spondylolysis)
Grade I	0–25 %
Grade II	25–50 %
Grade III	50–75 %
Grade IV	75–100 %
Grade V[a]	>100 % (spondyloptosis)

[a]Grades 0 and 5 are not part of original classification but added later and commonly used

involves the L5 nerve root and not the central canal. On exam, there can be a loss of lumbar lordosis, as well as limited flexion or extension, or pain with lumbar hyperextension. If advanced spondylolisthesis has occurred, the gait will be shortened in stride, with flexion at hips and knees due to hamstring contraction. Diagnosis of a pars defect or spondylolisthesis starts with radiographs with orthogonal views. The PA view can reveal a coexisting scoliosis due to muscle spasm, either coincidental or the result of asymmetric forward vertebral translation at the level of the spondolylisthesis. The lateral and oblique views are best to see a stress reaction or full defect. If radiographs are normal, a single-photon emission CT (SPECT) of lumbosacral spine with increased uptake in an otherwise intact-appearing pars, lamina, or pedicle is diagnostic of a stress reaction [27]. A thin-section CT with reverse gantry angle is the modality of choice for the bony anatomy of a spondylolysis; it can definitively assess cortical disruption, lysis, or sclerosis, as well as healing [28]. MRI has gradually replaced SPECT scans and CT as the best initial imaging modality as it will detect over 90 % of pars defects, reactive edema/stress responses, as well as disc herniations. MRI is always indicated if there are neurological symptoms that suggest the need to evaluate the surrounding soft tissues.

In a study by Micheli and Wood, spondylolytic stress fractures without cortical disruption in adolescent athletes have a chance to heal [29]. Healing potential of unilateral defects is greater than that of bilateral, and early treatment improved nonsurgical outcomes [30]. Early brace use has been shown to be superior to activity restriction alone, as well as to bracing following initial activity restriction. Patients with a spondylolytic defect consistent with true isthmic spondylolysis aim for pain relief and improvement of mobility over bony healing. Restricted activity, a short course of possible brace wearing, and physical therapy involving "sport specific exercise" activities have been shown to be effective [31]. High-grade spondylolisthesis does not respond as well to nonsurgical treatment. Surgical management is advised for symptomatic high-grade spondylolisthesis, though there is no data to support prophylactic treatment for asymptomatic spondylolisthesis of similar high grades. Other surgical indications include persistent pain despite a minimum of 6 months of conservative management.

When operative repair of a spondylolytic defect is required, the operative level determines the type of surgery that is to be performed. According to Hu et al. [32], when the spondylolytic defect is at L4 or above, a direct repair of the pars defect can be accomplished. Described techniques include direct screw fixation, tension wiring between the spinous process and transverse process, and screw with subliminal hook fixation. Karats et al. [33] in a comparison of direct compression screw versus pedicle screw with a subliminal hook showed no difference in clinical outcomes between the two techniques (Figs. 7.1 and 7.2). In a biomechanics study comparing the various fixation techniques, Fan et al. [34] demonstrated that the screw-rod-hook and screw-rod construct fixation techniques provided more stability than did the modified Scott and Buck techniques. In contrast with pars repair techniques at L4, when the defect occurs at L5, a posterior surgical fusion with instrumentation is indicated.

In tennis, the defects in the pars injuries are theorized to be more frequent with the modern tennis forehand stroke. The older style of play, in which the forehand

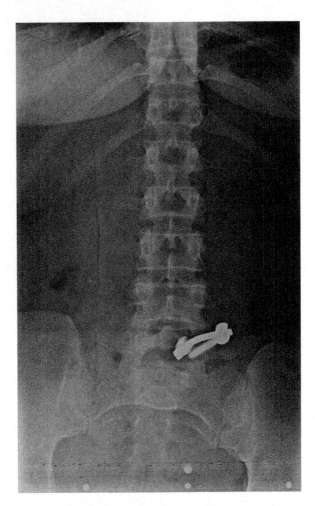

Fig. 7.1 AP radiograph demonstrating left-sided L5 pedicle screw with sublaminar hook

Fig. 7.2 Lateral
radiograph demonstrating
left-sided L5 pedicle screw
with sublaminar hook

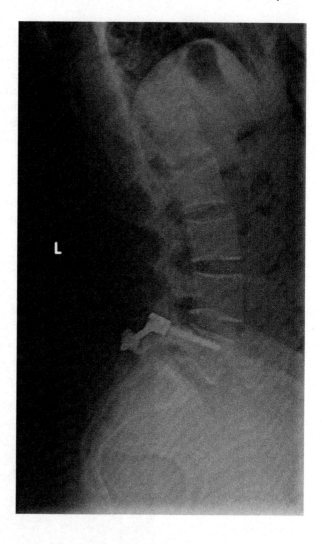

was hit with the stance lateral to the trajectory of the ball, resulted in an ascending torsion of legs through the trunk to the racket, and not overloading the pars. In the push to attain higher ball speeds and more top spin, a newer technique has been developed, where the forehand is hit from a stance facing the trajectory of the ball. In this position, the legs are partially flexed, and the hips are forced into sudden anteversion with forced hyperextension of the lumbar region, thereby placing increased stress on the pars region [32]. Additionally, as athletes are working to reach elite levels at earlier ages, an increase in this type of stroke occurs when spines are still developing, further precipitating the formation of a pars lesion. In a study of 66 young tennis athletes, with spondylosis divided into "developing" spondylosis with negative radiograph and positive SPECT, active spondylolysis with positive radiograph and SPECT, and established spondylolysis, with positive radiograph and negative SPECT, only three of eight patients with developing lysis who received a brace had healing of the defect, versus 7 of the remaining 19 cases of developing spondylolysis which healed with activity restriction and no brace. However, those with active lysis who wore a brace from diagnosis had lower mean time to decrease in pain [35]. In a study of 22 young athletes treated with surgical fusion for spondylolisthesis, 82 % returned to previous sport activity after an average of 7 months of rehabilitation [36]. Besides bracing, there are other nonoperative supplements treatment that have been used, such as external electrical stimulation, though the data is limited to case reports with poor descriptions of use and no clear link of electrical stimulation to the bony healing seen [37].

Disc Herniation

Symptomatic lumbar disc herniations in pediatric and adolescent patients are rare, though athletic activity involving excessive or repetitive axial loading is a significant risk factor [38]. Other risk factors relating to sports include poor conditioning, improper technique, and abrupt increases in training [39]. Thirty to 60 % of pediatric and teenage disc herniations are correlated with a trauma or sports-related injury event [40]. A symptomatic disc herniation most commonly presents with radiculopathy without back pain, and in young patients other skeletal diagnoses are often considered first; the time between onset and diagnosis is significantly longer in children and adolescents than adults [41].

Disc herniation occurs when the annulus fibrosis of the intervertebral disc is injured and permits the nucleus pulposus to exit the disc space into the central, lateral recess or peri-foraminal spaces of the spinal canal. The radicular symptoms are produced from compression of the traversing or exiting nerve roots by the herniated disc material. In general, pediatric herniations are most commonly paracentral [38]. The movements most inherent to the tennis stroke – rotation, flexion, and axial compression – are also those that are most correlated with disc herniation. It is important to ask the patient if there has been any recent increase or change in training prior to presentation, as well as if there are any specific activities that provoke pain. Symptoms of lumbar disc herniations are often worse in flexion. The straight leg raise, positive with pain radiating down the leg that occurs instead of back pain, is a sensitive test for lumbar pathology. In young patients, the SLR is positive in a majority of patients and crossed SLR in almost one-third [42]. However, tight hamstrings in children can be symptomatic of other pathologies, particularly spondylolysis or spondylolisthesis secondary to pars interarticularis lesions. L4–L5 and L5–S1 herniations constitute 90 % of symptomatic herniations, causing weakened great toe dorsiflexion and weakened ankle plantar flexion, respectively. However, disc bulges and herniations seen on MRI are not always symptomatic. Alyas et al. [42] showed that 30 % of adolescent tennis players with disc desiccation and bulging were entirely free of symptoms.

Plan X-rays can reveal a reactive scoliosis, caused by the body attempting to relieve compression on the affected nerve root, which is seen by the patient leaning to the contralateral side in order to widen the affected foramen. MRI is the gold standard for soft tissue diagnoses. CT and CT myelogram are best for bony detail another differential diagnoses, but do not illustrate the soft tissues as well.

Nonoperative treatment with rest, NSAIDs, muscle relaxants, and oral steroids are the first-line treatments. It has been shown, however, that younger patients do not do as well with conservative therapy [38]. Surgical options include open discectomy or microdiscectomy. In a series of 87 pediatric patients undergoing microdiscectomy following an average of 12.2 months of nonoperative therapy, overall outcomes were reported as good after 1 year [43]. Most elite tennis players return to their elite level of play after microdiscectomy. The average return time is 4–6 months.

Synovial Cysts

Synovial cysts, or ganglion cysts, are generally recognized to form from a defect in the joint capsule of a degenerative or unstable facet joint. They can occur throughout the spine, but are especially common in the lumbar spine. Though far more common in an older patient with degenerative osteoarthritis of the spine, they are thought to arise from joints in which there is abnormal motion or movement between the joint surfaces. The increase in stress placed on the more mobile segment of the lumbar spine, the L4–L5 and L5–S1 vertebrae, in the non-athlete is even more considerable in the active person. Tennis, with its repetitive twisting movements and rotational forces, likely only perseverates this pathophysiology. Likely mechanisms of the lumbar synovial cysts in young tennis athlete are micromotion or spondylolisthesis, which contributes atypical motion to the facet joints [44, 45].

Synovial cysts can be asymptomatic or present with symptoms of back pain, radicular compression, neurogenic claudication, and/or cauda equina syndrome that are not unheard of. MRI is the diagnostic modality of choice, as it accurately depicts their location and size in relation to the facet joints. It is typically low intensity on T1 and high intensity on T2, but that can be altered depending on the content of the fluid; these cysts can also be hemorrhagic if acute and therefore contain hemosiderin and have reduced signal intensity. The vast majority of these symptomatic cysts require surgical excision. Aspiration of the cyst has shown to be disappointing with regard to symptomatic relief and recurrence of symptoms. Many different surgical techniques are available, from simple excision alone to excision and fusion, depending on the surgeon and the underlying pathology that led to the development of the cyst. Developing a new cyst after initial surgical excision is rare, but reported in the literature [46]. Reported symptomatic cases in adolescents are rare and largely limited to case reports [44].

Facet Joint Arthropathy and Disc Degeneration

Degenerative discs and arthritis of the facet joints are more commonly seen in adults with symptoms of spinal stenosis and degenerative spondylolisthesis. Disc desiccation and degeneration can lead to loss of disc height, which results in infolding and buckling of ligamentum flavum. The ensuring abnormal mobility of lumbar spinal segments can lead to hypertrophic bony facets and facet joint capsules. Symptomatic compression of nerve roots can be caused by foramina compression from loss of disc height or lateral recess compression from enlarged facets. The altered ligamentous relationships of the spinal segment can also lead to degenerative spondylolisthesis, with resulting compression secondary to anterolisthesis of one vertebra on the one below it. This pathology is far more commonly seen in individuals over 50 years of age [47]. Signs of this in the pediatric or adolescent population are concerning for accelerated osteoarthritis of the spine, possibly due to excessive microtrauma to the ligaments and intervertebral disc-cartilaginous endplate interface. The long-term prognosis of these patients is not yet known, but it may lead to loss of athletic performance time or ability or even premature end to a playing career.

Other Entities

Besides the other, more chronic injuries discussed elsewhere in this chapter, there are several other injury entities described in the literature. As these are so rare, the diagnosis is commonly missed on initial exam and treatment. Disc herniation and disc degeneration were described earlier, but there are reports of acute intradiscal hematoma. The tennis player in question had buttock pain and the backhand stroke. He was treated for hip pathology, but symptoms returned with return ti play. Eventually, MRI revealed blood within the disc space, characterized by a hyperintense signal on T1. The player underwent serial MRIs over several years, with the hyperintense signal persisting until the disc in question became degenerative. The player was unable to return to play due to this injury [48].

Recently in the literature, Koehler et al. [49] described an acute apophyseal spinous process avulsion fracture in an elite athlete. A 12-year-old tennis player presented with 4 weeks of low back pain exacerbated by flexion and extension of the lumbar spine. Computed tomography (CT) was performed, revealing an avulsion fracture of the L5 spinous processes. The avulsion injury of the interspinous ligament was characterized by hypercellular fibrocartilage tissue, similar to that seen in severe Osgood-Schlatter's disease. The authors concluded that after 6 months of nonsurgical management for an athlete, surgical excision should be offered as an alternative.

Sacroiliac joint stress fractures are another rare cause of low back and buttock pain. In one published case report, the start of pain and eventual diagnosis stemmed from an increase in number of matches per week that he played. Radiographs were normal but MRI revealed significant bony edema at the SI joint. He was treated nonoperatively and with a dedicated stretching and strengthening program, and he was able to return to his sport [50]. This injury is likely due to a combination of vertical force from the stress of the body dissipating from spine into sacrum. There is probably also a role for the repetitive rotational repetition and changes in direction that make it a potential diagnosis.

Similar to the SI joint stress fractures, there are documented case series discussing sacral facet fractures. Clinical exam reveals patients with localized pain with back extension and hamstring tightness. The pain was severe enough to cease sport participation. MRI failed to diagnose the bony lesion eventually seen on CT. Fractures in the L5–S1 joint were appreciated. Patients were reported to have immediate pain relief and improvement of symptoms after surgical removal of fragment [51].

References

1. Muyor JM, Sanchez-Sanchez E, Sanz-Rivas D, et al. Spinal sagittal morphology in highly trained tennis players. J Sports Sci Med. 2013;12(3):588–93.
2. Pearcy M, Portek I, Shepherd J. Three-dimensional x-ray analysis of normal movement in the lumbar spine. Spine. 1984;9(3):294–7.
3. Bogduk N. Clinical anatomy of the lumbar spine and sacrum. 32nd ed. London, UK: Churchill Livingstone; 1997. p. 1–261.
4. McGill SM, Yingling VR, Peach JP. Three-dimensional kinematics and trunk muscle myoelectric activity in the elderly spine – a database compared to young people. Clin Biomech (Bristol, Avon). 1999;14(6):389–95.
5. White AA, Panjabi MM. Clinical biomechanics of the spine. 3rd ed. Philadelphia: Lippincott Williams & Wilkins; 1990.
6. Bergmark A. Stability of the lumbar spine. A study in mechanical engineering. Acta Orthop Scand Suppl. 1989;230:1–54.
7. Biering-Sorensen F. Physical measurements as risk indicators for low back trouble over a one year period. Spine (Phila Pa 1976). 1984;9(2):106–19.
8. Luoto S, Hellovaara M, Hurri H, et al. Static back endurance and the risk of low back pain. Clin Biomech (Bristol, Avon). 1995;10(6):323–4.
9. McGill SM, Grenier S, Bluhm M, et al. Previous history of LBP with work loss is related to lingering affects in biomechanical, physiological, personal, and psychosocial characteristics. Ergonomics. 2003;46(7):731–46.
10. Renkawitz T, Boluki D, Grifka J. The association of low back pain, neuromuscular imbalance, and trunk extension strength in athletes. Spine J. 2006;6(6):673–83.
11. Beach T, Parkinson R, Sothart P, et al. Effects of prolonged sitting on the passive flexion stiffness on the in vivo lumbar spine. Spine J. 2005;5(2):145–54.
12. Donatelli R, Dimond D, Holland M. Sport-specific biomechanics of spinal injuries in the athlete (throwing athletes, rotational sports, and contact-collision sports). Clin Sports Med. 2012;31(3):381–96.
13. Kong WZ, Goel VK, Gilbertson LG, et al. Effects of muscle dysfunction on lumbar spine mechanics: a finite element study based on a two motion segments model. Spine (Phila Pa 1976). 1996;21(19):2197–206. discussion 2206–7.
14. Kawasaki S, Imai S, Inaoka H, et al. The low lumbar spine moment and the axial rotational moment of a body during one-handed and double-handed backhand stroke in tennis. Int J Sports Med. 2005;26(8):617–21.

15. Campbell A, Straker L, O'Sullivan P, et al. Lumbar loading in the elite adolescent tennis serve: link to low back pain. Med Sci Sports Exerc. 2013;45(8):1562–8.
16. Abrams GD, Renstrom PA, Safran MR. Epidemiology of musculoskeletal injury in the tennis player. Br J Sports Med. 2012;46(7):492–8.
17. Hjelm N, Werner S, Renstrom P. Injury profile in junior tennis players: a prospective two year study. Knee Surg Sports Traumatol Arthrosc. 2010;18(6):845–50.
18. Pluim BM, Staal JB, Windler GE, et al. Tennis injuries: occurrence, aetiology, and prevention. Br J Sports Med. 2006;40(5):415–23.
19. Hutchinson MR, Laprade RF, Burnett 2nd QM, et al. Injury surveillance at the USTA Boys' Tennis Championships: a 6-yr study. Med Sci Sports Exerc. 1995;27(6):826–30.
20. Marks MJ, Haas SS, Wiesel SW. Low back pain in the competitive tennis players. Clin Sports Med. 1988;7(2):277–87.
21. Kibler B, Safran M. Tennis injuries. Med Sport Sci. 2005;48:120–37.
22. Fayssoux RS, Rhee JM. Spine injuries in sports. In: Rao R, editor. Orthopaedic knowledge update 4: spine. Rosemont: American Academy of Orthopaedic Surgeons; 2012. p. 263–72.
23. Rajeswaran G, Turner M, Gissane C, et al. MRI findings in the lumbar spines of asymptomatic elite junior tennis players. Skeletal Radiol. 2014;43(7):925–32.
24. Lundin O, Hellstrom M, Nilsson I, et al. Back pain and radiological changes in the thoraco-lumbar spine of athletes: a long-term follow up. Scand J Med Sci Sports. 2001;11(2):103–9.
25. Cavalier R, Herman MJ, Cheung EV, et al. Spondylolysis and spondylolisthesis in children and adolescents: I. Diagnosis, natural history and nonsurgical management. J Am Acad Orthop Surg. 2006;14(7):417–24.
26. Wiltse LL, Widell Jr EH, Jackson DW. Fatigue fracture: the basic lesion in isthmic spondylolisthesis. J Bone Joint Surg Am. 1975;57(1):17–22.
27. Lusins JO, Elting JJ, Cicoria AD, et al. SPECT evaluation of lumbar spondylolysis and spondylolisthesis. Spine (Phila Pa 1976). 1994;19(5):608–12.
28. Harvey CJ, Richenberg JL, Saifuddin A, et al. The radiological investigation of lumbar spondylolysis. Clin Radiol. 1998;53(10):723–8.
29. Micheli LJ, Wood R. Back pain in young athletes. Significant differences from adults in causes and patterns. Arch Pediatr Adolesc Med. 1995;149(1):15–8.
30. Sys J, Michielsen J, Bracke P, et al. Nonoperative treatment of active spondylolysis in elite athletes with normal X-ray findings: literature review and results of conservative treatment. Eur Spine J. 2001;10(6):498–504.
31. d'Hemecourt PA, Zurakowski D, Kriemler S, et al. Spondylolysis: returning the athlete to sports participation with brace treatment. Orthopedics. 2002;25(6):653–7.
32. Hu SS, Tribus CB, Diab M, et al. Spondylolisthesis and spondylolysis. Instr Course Lect. 2008;57:431–45.
33. Karatas AF, Dede O, Atanda AA, et al. Comparison of direct pars repair techniques of spondylolysis in pediatric and adolescent patients: pars compression screw versus pedicle screw-rod-hook. J Spinal Disord Tech. 2012 Oct 16. [Epub ahead of print]
34. Fan J, Yu GR, Liu F, et al. A biomechanical study on the direct repair of spondylolysis by different techniques of fixation. Orthop Surg. 2010;2(1):46–51.
35. Ruiz-Cotorro A, Balius-Matas R, Estruch-Massana AE, et al. Spondylolysis in young tennis players. Br J Sports Med. 2006;40(5):441–6. discussion 446.
36. Debnath UK, Freeman BJ, Gregory P, et al. Clinical outcome and return to sport after the surgical treatment of spondylolysis in young athletes. J Bone Joint Surg Br. 2003;85(2):244–9.
37. Stasinopoulos D. Treatment of spondylolysis with eternal electrical stimulation in young athletes: a critical literature review. Br J Sports Med. 2004;38(3):352–4.
38. Lavelle WF, Bianco A, Mason R, et al. Pediatric disk herniation. J Am Acad Orthop Surg. 2011;19(11):649–56.
39. Lawrence JP, Greene HS, Grauer JN. Back pain in athletes. J Am Acad Orthop Surg. 2006;14(13):726–35.

40. Papagelopoulos PJ, Shaughnessy WJ, Ebersold MJ, et al. Long-term outcome of lumbar discectomy in children and adolescents sixteen years of age or younger. J Bone Joint Surg Am. 1998;80(5):689–98.
41. Slotkin JR, Mislow JM, Day AL, et al. Pediatric disk disease. Neurosurg Clin N Am. 2007;18(4):659–67.
42. Alyas F, Turner M, Connell D. MRI findings in the lumbar spines of asymptomatic, adolescent, elite tennis players. Br J Sports Med. 2007;41(11):836–41. discussion 841.
43. Cahill KS, Dunn I, Gunnarsson T, et al. Lumbar microdiscectomy in pediatric patients: a large single-institution series. J Neurosurg Spine. 2010;12(2):165–70.
44. Gelabert-Gonzalez M, Prieto-Gonzalez A, Maria Santin-Amo J, et al. Lumbar synovial cyst in an adolescent: case report. Childs Nerv Syst. 2009;25(6):719–21.
45. Kalevski SK, Haritonov DG, Peev NA. Lumbar intraforaminal synovial cyst in young adulthood: case report and review of the literature. Global Spine J. 2014;4(3):191–6.
46. Shah RV, Lutz GE. Lumbar intraspinal synovial cysts: conservative management and review of the world's literature. Spine J. 2003;3(6):479–88.
47. Jenis LG. Lumbar spinal stenosis and degenerative spondylolisthesis. In: Rao R, editor. Orthopaedic knowledge update 4: spine. Rosemont: American Academy of Orthopaedic Surgeons; 2012. p. 329–38.
48. Baranto A, Hellstrom M, Sward L. Acute injury of intervertebral disc in an elite tennis player. Spine (Phila Pa 1976). 2010;35(6):E223–7.
49. Koehler SM, Rosario-Quinones F, Mayer J, et al. Understanding acute apophyseal spinous process avulsion injuries. Orthopedics. 2014;37(3):e317–21.
50. Silva RT, De Bortoli A, Laurino CF, et al. Sacral stress fracture: an unusual case of low back pain in an amateur tennis player. Br J Sports Med. 2006;40(5):460–1.
51. Skaggs DL, Avramis I, Myung K, et al. Sacral facet fractures in acute athletes. Spine (Phila Pa 1976). 2012;37(8):E514–7.

Chapter 8
Shoulder Injuries in the Young Tennis Athlete

Steven M. Koehler, Kristen M. Meier, and James N. Gladstone

Introduction

As a truly global sport, tennis is played by tens of millions worldwide, both for fun and competitively at all age levels. As a result, many young tennis players are playing at high levels and tennis-specific training often begins at an early age. Tennis is a stressful game to the shoulder. It requires multiple repetitions of large ranges of motions and high forces during all strokes. Because of the repetitive nature of the sport, the shoulder is often injured through overuse, especially in competitive, elite tennis athletes [46]. Early preventative measures can be taken in young tennis players to avoid specific injuries related to the sport. And early identification of injuries can allow for proper management and rehabilitation to give athletes the chance to not only continue playing but to do so at a high level.

Shoulder Anatomy

The shoulder has many unique and important anatomical characteristics that allow it to be the most mobile joint in the body. It is made up of three bones, the clavicle, the scapula, and the humerus, and three joints, the sternoclavicular, the acromioclavicular, and the glenohumeral; and it also is comprised of several associated muscles and ligaments (Fig. 8.1). The glenoid is relatively flat and its articular cavity is augmented by cartilage and a circumferential labrum. The large difference between the curvature and size of the humeral head compared with the glenoid requires both

S.M. Koehler, MD • K.M. Meier, MD • J.N. Gladstone, MD (✉)
Department of Orthopaedic Surgery, Mount Sinai Medical Center,
New York, NY, USA
e-mail: meier.kristen@gmail.com; James.Gladstone@mountsinai.org

© Springer International Publishing Switzerland 2016
A.C. Colvin, J.N. Gladstone (eds.), *The Young Tennis Player: Injury Prevention and Treatment,* Contemporary Pediatric and Adolescent Sports Medicine,
DOI 10.1007/978-3-319-27559-8_8

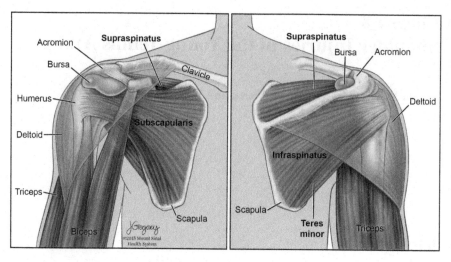

Fig. 8.1 The musculature of the shoulder (*left*) Anterior (*right*) Posterior

active stabilization by the deltoid and rotator cuff muscles and passive stabilization by the capsular ligaments and the increased depth of the glenoid conferred by the labrum.

Each joint has specific roles. The sternoclavicular joint helps to prevent displacement of the shoulder forward. It assists in shoulder abduction because the clavicle must elevate 40° to allow upward rotation of the scapula. At this joint, the clavicle will also move forward and backward to assist in flexion, extension, and internal and external rotation. There are anterior and posterior sternoclavicular ligaments that reinforce the joint capsule. There is an interclavicular ligament providing superior stability and a costoclavicular ligament attaching the inferior portion of the clavicle to the first rib and the costal cartilage. Dislocation of this joint is very rare. In adults the clavicle will usually fracture before the sternoclavicular joint dislocates. In people younger than 25 years of age, a dislocation of the sternoclavicular joint can occur from a fracture of the epiphyseal plate at the sternal end.

The acromioclavicular joint is the articulation of the acromion and distal clavicle. It is stabilized superiorly by the acromioclavicular ligament and posteriorly by the trapezius and deltoid muscle aponeuroses. The coracoclavicular ligaments also assist in stability of the joint. The joint is weak and sensitive to sprains. It assists in arm elevation by allowing the clavicle to rotate posteriorly.

The glenohumeral joint is well equipped for mobility. The ball and socket allows for three degrees of freedom. The first degree of freedom is the ability to flex and extend the shoulder. The second degree of freedom adds the ability to abduct and adduct. The two degrees working simultaneously result in the ability to circumduct the shoulder. The third degree of freedom is rotation. There are three glenohumeral ligaments: superior, middle, and inferior. The superior glenohumeral ligament limits inferior translation. The middle glenohumeral ligament limits external rotation at 45° of abduction, while the inferior glenohumeral ligament limits ER at 90° of abduction. There are three bursae in the shoulder that function to decrease friction: the subacromial, subdeltoid, and subscapular bursae, which may all interconnect and can become inflamed causing bursitis [66].

The superior shoulder suspensory complex is the system connecting the scapula to the axial skeleton (Fig. 8.2). It is extremely important biomechanically, with every component having its own function. It serves as a point of attachment for a variety of musculotendinous and ligamentous structures. It allows limited, but significant, movement to occur through the coracoclavicular ligament and the acromioclavicular articulation, and it maintains a normal, stable relationship between the upper extremity and the axial skeleton. It is composed of a bony and soft tissue ring connected to the trunk by superior and inferior struts. The ring includes the glenoid process, coracoid process, coracoclavicular ligament, distal clavicle, acromioclavicular joint, and acromion process. The superior strut is the middle third of the clavicle and the lateral part of the scapular body, and the medial part of the glenoid neck comprises the inferior strut [79].

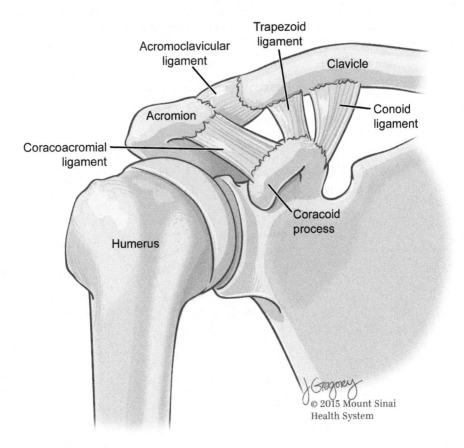

Fig. 8.2 The bony anatomy of the shoulder

The developmental anatomy of the shoulder is predictable and knowledge of it is critical to the appropriate diagnosis of bony injuries of the skeletally immature athlete's shoulder [78]. The initial ossification center, the proximal medial humeral epiphysis, becomes radiographically apparent at 4 months of age (Fig. 8.3). The greater tuberosity secondary ossification center appears between 6 and 18 months, and the lesser tuberosity shortly thereafter. The greater tuberosity and proximal humeral ossification centers fuse to form the proximal humeral epiphysis by age 4–7 years. Closure of this physis usually is complete by ages 14–16 in girls and in boys by ages 17–21. The clavicle has secondary ossification centers at the sternal and acromial ends. The secondary center of ossification of the acromial end is a thin epiphysis that fuses to the distal clavicular metaphysis by age 19 years. The secondary ossification center of the sternal clavicle appears between 15 and 18 years of age and fuses at 20–25 years of age. The scapula has seven secondary ossification centers, two of which form the acromion that develop between 14 and 16 years of age, fuse by age 19 years, and fuse to the scapular spine by age 25 years. Failure of acromial fusion to each other or to the scapula results in an os acromiale, the type depends on which centers fail to fuse. There are two ossification centers of the scapular body. Three ossification centers at the base, middle, and tip of the process form the coracoid. Fusion of coracoid ossification centers is complete by age 18 years.

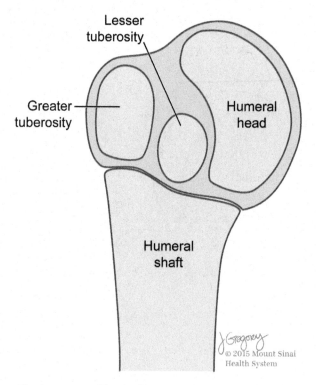

Fig. 8.3 The ossification centers of the shoulder

Tennis Biomechanics

Large demands are placed on the shoulder (glenohumeral, acromioclavicular, and sternoclavicular joints) in terms of the range of motion, loads, and velocity required during tennis [47]. In order to play tennis, the glenohumeral joint must have an arc of 160–180° of motion (internal + external rotation) and the highest point of abduction is between 140 and 160° [25]. The velocity of the glenohumeral joint goes from 0°/s in external rotation at late cocking, just prior to serve, to 1140–1715°/s in internal rotation during the serve. The 1-hand backhand stroke generates rotational velocities up to 900°/s, whereas the open stance forehand generates 280°/s [25]. These result in arm velocities ranging from 34 miles/h to 72 miles/h. This extraordinary acceleration results in glenohumeral joint loads up to two times the patient's bodyweight.

In addition to the incredible velocities and range of motion experienced by the athlete's shoulder, the torques generated in the serve are equally impressive [24]. These torques have been reported as high as 65 Nm at maximal external rotation and 70 Nm at acceleration to ball impact. Torques greater than 50 Nm are considered supraphysiologic and therefore a potentially significant factor in producing injury, particularly overload injuries [120].

As the young tennis player continues to train, the musculoskeletal system adapts to sport-specific demands via altered flexibility, strength, muscle balance, and endurance [11, 14, 29, 47–49, 51, 113]. Flexibility measurements in tennis players were significantly lower in sit-and-reach, dominant shoulder internal rotation and non-dominant shoulder internal rotation tests compared to non-throwing, non-tennis athletes. Tennis players were also shown to be more flexible in the external rotation of both shoulders [48]. These flexibility differences suggest that adaptations take place in response to the repetitive, short-duration, high-velocity, and highly tensile demands of tennis. While these adaptations could be considered as "normal," efforts to control the high forces generated by this sport create biomechanical inefficiencies and cause functional alterations that decrease optimal performance and increase injury risk [11, 51].

In addition to the repetitive demands on the shoulder, tennis also requires explosive movement patterns and highly intensive maximal-effort concentric and eccentric muscular work. The tennis serve and forehand strokes gain power from internal rotation at the shoulder. The internal rotators must tighten to accelerate while the external rotators must eccentrically contract during follow-through of the stroke or serve [23].

Groundstrokes require predominantly horizontal actions at the shoulder, using a combination of abduction and external rotation for the forehand backswing and backhand follow-through and a combination of adduction and internal rotation for the forehand forward swing and backhand backswing.

The overhead tennis serve is often related to throwing with the uses of combinations of horizontal and vertical movements. The stages of a tennis serve are similar to that of an overhead throwing athlete, with similar motions. Tennis serves are divided into three distinct phases, preparation, acceleration, and follow-through, and these three phases can be further subdivided into eight stages [56]. The preparation phase is subdivided into (1) start, (2) release, (3) loading, and (4) cocking. The acceleration phase is subdivided into (5) acceleration and (6) contact. And lastly, the follow-through phase is subdivided into (7) deceleration and (8) finish (Fig. 8.4). As in throwing, the greatest stress on the racquet arm is during the cocking, acceleration, deceleration, and finish phases. Horizontal abduction and external rotation occur during cocking. High torque forces and glenohumeral joint compressive loads are generated. High anterior shear force and large internal rotation and abduction torques are produced during this phase. Periscapular muscles stabilize the scapula and position the glenoid. The deltoid and the rotator cuff work synergistically to elevate the arm and maintain glenohumeral congruency. Acceleration begins with the initiation of humeral internal rotation. Very high angular velocities, torques, and joint compressive forces occur with scapular retraction and depression into the loading phase. During the acceleration phase, scapular elevation, horizontal abduction, and shoulder extension move the arm toward contact. Internal rotation, shoulder extension, and adduction complete the follow-through phase. The muscles of the rotator cuff play a vital role in stabilizing the humeral head in the glenoid during

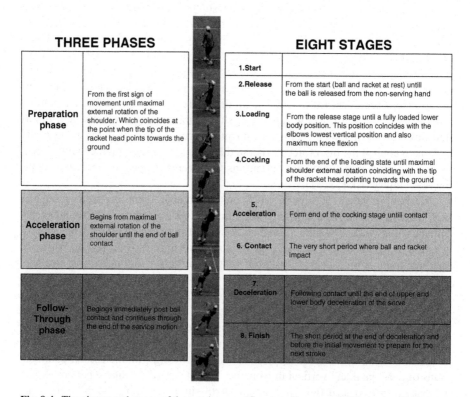

THREE PHASES		EIGHT STAGES	
		1. Start	
Preparation phase	From the first sign of movement until maximal external rotation of the shoulder. Which coincides at the point when the tip of the racket head points towards the ground	2. Release	From the start (ball and racket at rest) untill the ball is released from the non-serving hand
		3. Loading	From the release stage until a fully loaded lower body position. This position coincides with the elbows lowest vertical position and also maximum knee flexion
		4. Cocking	From the end of the loading state until maximal shoulder external rotation coinciding with the tip of the racket head pointing towards the ground
Acceleration phase	Begins from maximal external rotation of the shoulder until the end of ball contact	5. Acceleration	Form end of the cocking stage untill contact
		6. Contact	The very short period where ball and racket impact
Follow-Through phase	Begings immediately post ball contact and continues through the end of the service motion	7. Deceleration	Following contact until the end of upper and lower body deceleration of the serve
		8. Finish	The short period at the end of deceleration and before the initial movement to prepare for the next stroke

Fig. 8.4 The phases and stages of the tennis serve (Courtesy Kovacs and Ellenbecker [56])

all tennis movements, but they are critical during the acceleration and follow-through phases of the serve. The muscles of the rotator cuff aid in power production during acceleration and provide eccentric strength to help slow down the arm after contact during deceleration. It has been reported that during the explosive internal rotation of the serve, shoulder rotation can reach speeds from 1,074 to 2,300°/s. After contact, deceleration has to occur through eccentric contraction of the rotator cuff and related musculature. The posterior rotator cuff and periscapular muscles are active during this phase. At the professional level, male players reach speeds on the serve close to 140 miles per hour (225 km/h). Thus, proper conditioning of the shoulder musculature is critical.

Tennis volleys require smaller muscle and joint movements than either ground-strokes or serves. For a forehand volley, slight external rotation and slight adduction followed by abduction of the shoulder allow the player to complete the stroke. The backhand volley involves slight internal rotation and adduction followed by slight external rotation and abduction of the shoulder.

There are glenohumeral and scapulothoracic alterations described in elite tennis players. In a study performed in 59 elite adolescent players, researchers found that players older than 16 years old showed less scapular rotation on the dominant side at 90 and 180°. The presence of sufficient upward rotation during overhead movements has been suggested as vital to injury-free performance by clearing the acromion from the underlying subacromial structures.

Shoulder Pathology in Tennis: Injury Patterns, Incidence, and Background

In high-level players under 18 years of age, injury rates have been estimated to be anywhere from 2 to 20 injuries per 1000 h of tennis played [4, 35, 102]. Pluim et al. examined the incidence of tennis injuries in players of all levels and reported a range of 0.04–3.0 injuries per 1000 h played [84]. An interesting trend often reported is that lower extremity injuries frequently present acutely and upper extremity injuries manifest themselves chronically [3, 84, 85]. When studies concerning injuries in adolescent elite national tennis players are looked at collectively, the lower extremity is found to be where most injuries occur (31–67 %), followed closely by the upper extremity (20–49 %) and finally the trunk (3–21 %). The most common upper extremity injuries involve the shoulder and elbow. In a study of youth high-level tennis players aged 12–19, 24 % reported shoulder pain [62].

Data from a USTA survey showed that 25–35 % of tennis players involved in the boys' and girls' national championships had prior or current shoulder pain. Of those male athletes who reported shoulder pain, 38 % experienced anterior shoulder pain, 30 % experienced posterior, and 32 % noted both anterior and posterior shoulder pain. Of the female athletes who reported shoulder pain, 56 % experienced anterior shoulder pain, 15 % experienced posterior, and 31 % experienced both anterior and posterior shoulder pain.

The most common types of injury in tennis players of all ages are muscle strains and ligament sprains secondary to overuse. This is a failure of the body to respond to chronic, repetitive, microtraumatic overload. Children and adolescents are at particular risk for sport-related overuse injuries as a result of improper technique, training errors, improper equipment, and muscle weakness and imbalance. However, increasing numbers of chronic overuse injuries in young athletes may be related to limited recovery from longer competitive seasons and year-round training [5].

Multiple studies have examined player-specific risk factors for injury. Age and sex were studied by Jayanthi et al. [43] and there was no correlation with injuries. Other investigators have also corroborated these findings [117]. Currently, as in many other overhead sports, the volume of play is correlated with an increased injury rate. The overall injury rate has been reported to increase for individuals playing more than 3 h per week [85]. It seems intuitive that differing skill levels would also have differing rates of injuries. However, the overall incidence and prevalence of injury do not differ [43]. Despite these findings, studies have reported differences in the stresses and forces experienced between skill levels. Compared to more proficient players, less experienced players are subjected to higher vibration loads. As one would expect, novice players have more variability in the contact point of the ball on the strings, as well as differing grip forces [33, 114]. Reduced grip forces allow for decreased vibration being transferred from the racquet to the arm, thereby lowering the rate of upper extremity injuries [33]. The paradoxical result that the incidence and prevalence of injuries are no different among skill levels may be accounted for by the increased volume of play in the semiprofessional and professional groups. Lastly, while studies have examined the role of grip position in relation to the biomechanics and loads transmitted to the wrist, there is no study examining the impact on the shoulder. Likewise there have been no studies to determine the effect of arm vibration on injury rate or severity.

Physical Examination

Physical examination of the shoulder in the skeletally immature athlete must also include a complete examination of the cervical spine and the uninvolved shoulder. Examination of the young tennis player's shoulder is identical to that of the adult shoulder and should include inspection, palpation, evaluation of range of motion, stability testing, and special tests such as impingement signs. Determination of generalized ligamentous laxity is important because increased glenohumeral translation in a setting of generalized hyperlaxity is common in skeletally immature patients. Differentiating pathologic laxity from generalized ligamentous laxity can be difficult and may depend on demonstrating laxity asymmetry, which is the reason it is important to compare both range of motion and extent of translation with the opposite shoulder. It is also important to recognize adaptive changes that occur in the tennis player's dominant shoulder over time (increased external rotation, decreased internal rotation). Additionally, it is not uncommon to develop upper extremity, shoulder girdle, and paraspinous physiologic hemihypertrophy. Additionally, and particularly in players with overuse injuries, the kinetic chain should be followed distally to ensure that overstress on the shoulder has not been caused by a problem in the foot, knee, hip or back.

Examination should be thorough and ideally occur in a patient without a shirt on or in a sports bra for the best assessment of the shoulder. During inspection, an examiner may notice excessive thoracic kyphosis or cervical lordosis. Asymmetry (medial or lateral winging), atrophy, or hypertrophy of certain parts of the shoulder can be visible on inspection. Palpation of bony prominences as well as soft tissue structures is necessary including the borders of the scapula, sternoclavicular joint, acromioclavicular joint, coracoid process, greater and lesser tuberosities of the humerus, subacromial bursa, supraclavicular fossa, long head of the biceps tendon, the trapezius, the levator scapulae, the rhomboids, the rotator cuff muscles, and the deltoid. The shoulder range of motion must be assessed in all planes: forward elevation, external rotation at the side and at 90° of abduction, internal rotation to a vertebral height, and abduction. These should be tested on both sides.

A complete neurovascular exam must also be documented by the examiner. Important sensory dermatomes to be evaluated include the axillary, musculocutaneous, medial brachial and antebrachial cutaneous, median, radial, and ulnar nerve distributions. The important muscles to isolate and test include the rotator cuff, deltoid, biceps, triceps, extensor pollicis longus, flexor digitorum profundus, and the dorsal interossei. A vascular exam to assess the brachial, radial, and ulnar arteries should be performed without exception. Once the initial exam is performed, the provocative tests listed in Table 8.1 should be performed to help rule in or rule out specific conditions or injuries.

Imaging

Plain radiography is the primary imaging modality for evaluating sports injuries to the shoulder. A standard trauma series should be obtained in all patients presenting with pain: anteroposterior (AP) radiograph of the shoulder, AP radiograph of the glenohumeral joint (Grashey view), axillary radiograph, and scapular Y radiograph. Additional views can be obtained as necessary: apical oblique, Velpeau, West Point axillary, Stryker notch, Zanca and Serendipity. Additionally, when imaging skeletally immature patients, it is often helpful to obtain views of the contralateral side.

Depending on the history, physical exam, and radiographs, advanced imaging may be indicated. Magnetic resonance imaging (MRI) is a vital diagnostic tool in many shoulder pathologies. MRI provides an unparalleled examination of the soft tissues. Additionally it provides multiplanar imaging capabilities. In the skeletally immature athlete, MRI can afford imaging of the growing physis, musculotendinous units, ligaments, marrow spaces, and more. Not all studies are equal, however, and

Table 8.1 Shoulder Physical Examination Provocative Tests

Rotator cuff	Provocative test	Description	Positive test	Possible etiologies for positive tests
	Jobe's test/empty can test	Abduct arm to 90° in the scapular plane, internally rotate. Examiner will press down on arm while patient attempts to maintain position	Pain; arm falls to side	Subacromial bursitis, supraspinatus weakness or tear (if arm falls down)
	Drop sign (Codman's)	Elevate arm in scapular plane to 90°. Patient is then asked to slowly lower the arm	pain, weakness; arm falls to side	Supraspinatus weakness, injury, or tear
	External rotation lag sign	Fully externally rotate shoulder with elbow flexed to 90°	Arm moves into internal rotation	Infraspinatus weakness, injury, or tear
	Hornblower's sign	Abduct arm to 90°, externally rotate. Patient asked to maintain position	Arm moves into internal rotation	Teres minor weakness, injury, or tear
	Internal rotation lag sign	Elevate and extend arm to 20°; fully internally rotate shoulder as examiner is holding wrist and supporting elbow. Patient asked to maintain position	Arm drifts to neutral	Subscapularis weakness, injury, or tear (description of test unclear)
	Increased passive external rotation	Externally rotate both shoulders	One shoulder has increased external rotation	Subscapularis weakness, injury, or tear
	Gerber lift-off test	Internally rotate shoulder and place hand at lumbar region with palm facing outward; ask patient to lift hand away from back	Inability to perform test	Subscapularis weakness, injury, or tear usually in the inferior portion of the muscle. Test can be confounded by other muscle injuries
	Belly press	Internally rotate shoulder and place palm on abdomen	Elbow falls to side	Subscapularis weakness, injury, or tear usually in the superior portion of the muscle

Impingement	Neer test	Internally rotate shoulder and flex arm upward while examiner stabilizes scapula	Pain over coracoacromial arch	Rotator cuff tendinitis. Impingement of supraspinatus tendon or long head of the biceps. Other etiologies cause positive findings: stiff joint, osteoarthritis, instability, bone lesions
	Hawkin's test	Flex shoulder to 90° and bend elbow to 90°. The examiner then internally rotates the shoulder	Pain over coracoacromial arch	Rotator cuff tendinitis. Impingement of supraspinatus tendon or long head of the biceps
	Crossover test	Flex shoulder to 90°, internally rotate shoulder, while examiner adducts arm	Pain over coracoacromial arch or at AC joint	Impingement of supraspinatus tendon or long head of the biceps. Also positive with AC joint pathology
Labral injuries	O'Brien's test, active compression test	Flexion of shoulder to 90°, adduct to 30–45°, and maximally internally rotate shoulder. The forearm is pronated while examiner places a downward force. Repeat with supination of forearm	Pain with pronation but not supination	SLAP tear. Also positive with AC joint and biceps pathology
	Crank test	Abduct shoulder to 90°. Examiner holds arm and passively rotates shoulder while placing an axial load on joint	Clicking or pain in glenohumeral joint	SLAP lesion or tear
	Anterior slide	Patient places hands on hips while examiner has one hand anteriorly on shoulder and posteriorly on elbow. Examiner then places an anterosuperiorly directed force with the patient resisting	Pain at anterosuperior shoulder, a pop or click, or reproduction of symptoms	Impingement of superior labrum between humeral head and glenoid
	Clunk test/labral test	Patient lies supine while examiner places one hand posterior to shoulder and one hand around proximal forearm. Examiner then abducts the arm over the head while placing an anterior force on the humeral head and externally rotating humerus with distal hand	Clunk or grinding sensation at glenohumeral joint	Labral tear. This test will cause apprehension if a patient has anterior instability

(continued)

Table 8.1 (continued)

Rotator cuff	Provocative test	Description	Positive test	Possible etiologies for positive tests
Biceps brachii	Speed's test	Shoulder flexed to 90, forearm supinated with an extended elbow. Examiner places downward force while patient tries to flex arm	Pain in the area of the bicipital groove	Biceps tendonitis
	Yergason's test	Patient flexes elbow to 90° with arm at side. The patient then attempts supination against resistance by the examiner	Pain in the area of the bicipital groove	Biceps tendonitis
	Booth and Marvel test/transverse humeral ligament test	Patient flexes elbow to 90° with arm at side. Examiner uses one hand to gently pull downward traction and externally rotate the shoulder. The examiner's other hand should be in the area of the bicipital groove	Subluxation, pain, popping, or clicking in the area of the bicipital groove	Subluxing biceps tendon
	Ludington's test	Patient clasps hands and places on top of head. Then the patient alternately contracts and relaxes the biceps while the examiner places hands on shoulders	Inability of examiner to palpate long head of biceps tendon	Ruptured biceps tendon (long head)
AC joint	AC shear test	Examiner places hand over shoulder joint (acromion and coracoid processes) and compresses	Pain	AC or CC ligament tears
	Active compression test	See above	Pain with pronation but not supination	AC joint pathology. Also positive for SLAP tear

Anterior instability				
	Anterior load and shift	Patient lies supine and flexes shoulder to 90 degrees and abducts 40–60°. Examiner places axial load to the humerus with anteriorly and posteriorly directed forces	Increased anterior translation compared to contralateral side	Anterior instability
	Apprehension and relocation	1. Patient lies supine. Examiner brings arm to 90° of abduction and fully externally rotates 2. Examiner places hand on anterior shoulder and applies a posterior force on the humeral head	Positive if patient first experiences a sense of instability and if the second movement causes elimination of the instability	Anterior instability, also indicative of internal impingement with a posterosuperior labral tear and/or posterosuperior partial tearing of the cuff
	Anterior release	Patient lies supine. Examiner brings shoulder to abduction and external rotation while placing hand on the humeral head to keep the shoulder reduced. Then the examiner removes that hand	If the patient has instability when hand is removed	Anterior instability
	Anterior drawer	Examiner stabilizes scapula while applying an anteriorly directed force on humeral head with contralateral hand	If there is increased translation compared to the contralateral side	Anterior instability

(continued)

Table 8.1 (continued)

Rotator cuff	Provocative test	Description	Positive test	Possible etiologies for positive tests
Posterior instability	Posterior load and shift	Same technique as anterior load and shift	Increased posterior translation compared to contralateral side	Posterior instability
	Jerk test	Patient sits up with shoulder flexed to 90° and internally rotated to 90°. Examiner places axial and posterior force to humerus	Clunk or pain	Posterior instability
	Posterior drawer	Same technique as anterior drawer with a posteriorly directed force	If there is increased translation compared to the contralateral side	Posterior instability
	Posterior stress test	Patient flexes shoulder while adducting and internally rotating shoulder. Examiner places a posteriorly directed force	Pain, sense of instability	Posterior instability
Multidirectional instability	Sulcus sign	Patient stands with arms at side. Examiner pulls inferiorly on arm	Sulcus forms between superior aspect of humeral head and acromion	Multidirectional instability

meticulous acquisition, dedicated surface coils, tailored protocols with thin slices, small field of view and large imaging matrices are critical to obtaining high-quality studies. When labral tears are suspected, an MR arthrogram can be extremely helpful.

Computed tomography (CT) is often avoided in skeletally immature patients due to the radiation dose. CT does have a significant radiation dose and this should always be a consideration [7]. However, CT often provides vital and irreplaceable detail of complex bony injuries that conventional roentgenograms cannot. In difficult decisions such as whether or not a patient needs an operative intervention, the fine bony detail of a CT scan can provide this answer. Therefore, in the proper patient, a medically indicated CT scan far outweighs any risk of radiation.

General Rehabilitation

Rehabilitation of the shoulder must be tailored to the specific injury or surgery. In general, it consists of controlled recovery of a complete range of motion, followed by a comprehensive strengthening program focusing on the rotator cuff and periscapular musculature. Optimal rehabilitation and improved performance of the dynamic stabilizers decrease the stresses on passive restraints. Rehabilitation protocols must include posterior capsular stretching and strengthening exercises for the rotator cuff and periscapular muscles including concentric and eccentric exercises and plyometrics. The final phase of shoulder rehabilitation is an interval-hitting program that provides a graduated return to the stresses of tennis. An appropriate return to a tennis program emphasizes reestablishing or developing proper serve and stroke mechanics. We recommend partnering with both the athlete's tennis coach and a physical therapist to custom-tailor the rehabilitation program.

Rotator Cuff Pathology

The shoulder is the most commonly affected part of the upper extremity, with rotator cuff inflammation being one of the most common injuries in tennis players of all levels. The rotator cuff is a group of muscles and tendons that stabilize the shoulder and allow it to be the most mobile joint in the body. The rotator cuff muscles maintain the humeral head inside the glenoid cavity.

In addition to stabilizing the glenohumeral joint and controlling humeral head translation, the rotator cuff muscles also perform multiple functions, including abduction, internal rotation, and external rotation of the shoulder. The infraspinatus and subscapularis have significant roles in scapular plane shoulder abduction generating forces that are two to three times greater than the force produced by the supraspinatus muscle. However, the supraspinatus is more effective for general shoulder abduction because of its moment arm. The anterior portion of the supraspinatus tendon can handle significantly greater load and stress than the middle and posterior portion and seems to perform the main functional role [41]. Adaptations to the scapula discussed in a future section of the chapter in tennis players also can increase the risk of developing rotator cuff injuries.

Rotator cuff inflammation usually occurs as a result of chronic repetitive hitting and overhead serving [11]. Classic symptoms include point tenderness over the anterolateral acromion, a positive impingement sign, glenohumeral subluxation, and a positive anterior slide test. In contrast to older players with rotator cuff pathology, commonly attributable to impingement and degenerative changes, the young player's symptoms are more likely to be secondary to instability of the glenohumeral joint [76]. A loss of strength in the external rotators and scapular stabilizers accompanied by a loss of flexibility in the internal rotators has been associated with instability [44, 45, 52]. In more affected individuals, the posterior capsule, shoulder external rotators, and scapular stabilizers become fatigued, followed by superior and/or anterior glenohumeral translation due to the pull of the deltoid and trapezius during overhead arm motion.

When evaluating the shoulder, therefore, flexibility, strength, and instability must be tested. Treatment of rotator cuff inflammation should begin conservatively, with rest, avoidance of overhead arm activity, application of ice, and anti-inflammatory medications. Improving flexibility and strength starts with exercises for the scapular stabilizers followed by exercises for the rotator cuff after 2–3 weeks. By 6–8 weeks, most of the symptoms should be resolved and functional deficits should have been corrected [11].

Rotator cuff tears are much less commonly found in skeletally immature athletes than in adults. Young overhead athletes, however, do experience tendonitis and subacromial impingement [115]. Overuse injuries are increasing and are responsible for up to 70 % of visits to the pediatric sports medicine clinics [36].

Rotator cuff tears in tennis players can be repaired successfully, and the athlete has a good chance of returning to previous level of play. Studies discussing return to play after rotator cuff repair in youth tennis athletes could not be found by the authors. McCann and Bigliani [73] reported on the results of rotator cuff repair and acromioplasty in 23 adult tennis players. There were eight small tears (<1 cm), five moderate tears (1–3 cm), two large tears (3–5 cm), and eight massive tears (>5 cm). At a mean follow-up of 42 months, the authors reported that 19 patients (83 %) achieved a good to excellent result and were able to return to their presymptomatic level of play without pain. Ground strokes were not permitted before 6 months and overhead serves were restricted until 1 year following the operation.

Bicipital Tendonitis

Inflammation of the long head of the biceps tendon is a common cause of shoulder pain. While uncommonly reported in adolescents, it has been reported in adolescent tennis players [108]. The diagnosis often accompanies impingement and/or instability. The pain is frequently located on the anterior face of the shoulder and is exacerbated by active anterior elevation and external rotation. The pathophysiology of bicipital tendonitis likely occurs during the cocking stage: the shoulder is hyperextended, externally rotated, and abducted with a flexed elbow. The anterior structures are under tension which can lead to inflammation in the long head. Once diagnosed, it is important to ask the athlete whether they have recently changed their racquet; had previous shoulder pain, trauma, or instability; or increased their frequency or duration of play. Occasionally tendonitis can be seen related to equipment, in which case the athlete should cease play with the offending racquet and/or string tension. If none of these causes can be attributed to the tendonitis, then it is likely that the athlete has technical errors when cocking and an in-depth strokemechanics analysis is recommended. In the event of isolated bicipital tendonitis, we recommend cessation from play and rest for 4–6 weeks. In the event of a partial tear, 3–5 months of rest is needed for recovery [108].

SLAP Tear/Labral Pathology

Labral and/or biceps anchor injuries are rare in preadolescents, but superior labrum anterior to posterior (SLAP) lesions do occur in adolescent overhead athletes [39, 40, 55, 83]. As in adults, the athlete commonly presents with pain at the extreme of external rotation occurring in the cocking phase or with pain at follow-through. It is thought that the forces during the late coking and acceleration phases of throwing create a "peel-back" phenomenon that lead to SLAP tears [9, 100]. Clinical examination may demonstrate a positive O'Brien's sign, but physical examination is often nonspecific [32]. Plain radiographs are normal. MR arthrogram is the diagnostic test of choice and an abduction external rotation (ABER) view can further enhance the findings. SLAP tears are extremely unusual in adolescents and treatment should initially be conservative. If unsuccessful, surgical treatment is similar to adults. Whether a lesion is debrided or repaired is based on the Snyder classification [105]. Type I lesions rarely require treatment. Type III lesions are debrided. Type II lesions are the most common clinically significant SLAP tears. These are characterized by the detachment of the superior labrum/biceps anchor from the glenoid. Unstable type II lesions should be repaired. Treatment of type IV tears depends on the extent of biceps tendon involvement. When less than 30 % of the biceps is involved, type IV lesions are treated with repair of the labrum and biceps debridement. Greater than 30 % in a young patient is generally treated with biceps tenodesis and labral repair.

However, surgical results do not necessarily translate to a return to high performance in overhead athletes. Ide et al. in 2005 found only 75 % of overhead athletes were able to return to their preinjury level of play, despite 90 % of patients achieving a good or excellent result [38]. Another series by Kim et al. looked at 34 patients, with an average follow-up of 33 months from surgery [54]. They reported 94 % good to excellent results, with 91 % reporting a full return to normal function.

However, only 22 % of patients were able to return to the same level of sporting activity. Additionally, Cohen et al. analyzed the ability of throwers to return to professional baseball after a SLAP repair [75]. Twenty-two professional baseball players underwent arthroscopic repair of SLAP tears by a variety of the most experienced sports shoulder surgeons in the United States; all underwent the same focused, structured postoperative rehabilitation under the guidance of experienced professional baseball athletic trainers. In spite of this, only 32 % were able to return to the same level of professional baseball. No difference was identified in outcome from one surgeon to another or from pitcher to position player. Neuman et al. evaluated patients who underwent arthroscopic repair of a type II SLAP tear and who participated in overhead athletics, including many at an elite level [75]. Of the 30 patients in the study, the mean ASES score was 87.9, with 93.3 % of patients stating they were either satisfied or very satisfied with the results of their surgery at an average of 3.5 years' follow-up. The results were similar to other studies where the ASES scores were comparable among the patients regardless of their sport or position, and all patients reported high satisfaction rates with their outcome following surgery. Despite these positive results, throwing athletes continue to report decreased ability to return to their pre-injury level of play.

In the face of this data, we recommend nonoperative treatment of SLAP tears in elite young tennis players first and foremost. Only if the athlete has failed multiple attempts at conservative treatment and complains of an inability to play or persistently decreased performance should surgical intervention be considered.

Glenohumeral Internal Rotation Deficit

Glenohumeral internal rotation deficit (GIRD) is an often diagnosed problem in overhead sports players such as tennis, volleyball, baseball, and swimming athletes. Originally, the etiology was thought to be due to progressive lengthening of the inferior glenohumeral ligament; however, more recent studies have shown that the loss in glenohumeral internal rotation is due to tightness in the posteroinferior capsule due to repetitive microtrauma [2, 10]. Tehranzadeh et al. and Thomas et al. have shown posterior capsule thickening in athletes with GIRD using magnetic resonance imaging (MRI) and ultrasound, respectively. Posterior capsule tightness creates obligatory anterior and superior translation of the humeral head and loss of internal rotation. Abnormal humeral translation is not the result of ligament insufficiency or laxity but rather asymmetrical capsular tightness [110]. Most athletes are initially asymptomatic even with significant deficits. In a study of 54 asymptomatic tennis players and swimmers compared to controls, tennis players were found to have a mean GIRD of 23.9° versus 12° in swimmers and 4.9° in controls [107]. Athletes with this deficit have been shown to develop internal impingement and pain. Ideally, patients should be treated nonoperatively and conservative rehabilitation programs specific to this entity have been developed including but not limited to the supine sleeper stretch [70].

In a study of 22 patients with internal impingement, GIRD, and posterior shoulder tightness (ages 17–62), patients were prescribed physical therapy three times per week for approximately 7 weeks in addition to a home exercise program. All patients significantly improved. 10 patients had complete resolution of symptoms of pain from internal impingement while 12 had minor residual symptoms [109]. In a study of 62 overhead athletes aged 18–30 years with GIRD of greater than 15° at baseline compared to the non-dominant side, athletes were randomized to a 6-week stretching program versus the control group which had no intervention. The athletes had to be asymptomatic for at least 6 months to be included in the study. Due to the risk of subacromial impingement with GIRD, the acromiohumeral distance was also measured in these patients and compared at the beginning and end of the treatment program. The mean change in GIRD in the treatment group was 24.7° and the acromiohumeral distance decreased slightly 0.4 mm, 0.5 mm, and 0.6 mm at 0, 45, and 60°, respectively [69]. This study in addition to others shows that GIRD is at least partially reversible [50, 67].

In patients with intractable GIRD leading to chronic impingement and pain, surgical management includes arthroscopic posterior capsular release. In a study of 47 overhead athletes (ages 15–35) who underwent arthroscopic capsular release, 16 had no concomitant lesions and were retrospectively reviewed with a follow-up of at least 2 years. Fourteen had complete resolution of pain. In terms of throwing power, 90–100 % recovery was achieved in 11 patients, 70–80 % in 4, and 50–60 % in 1 [119].

Scapular Dyskinesis

"Tennis shoulder" refers to a drooping, internally rotated shoulder caused by long-term overhead arm use contributing to generalized laxity of the shoulder capsule and musculature [88]. The findings with tennis shoulder are not commonly reported in adolescents [49]. This is likely because the young shoulder has not yet experienced enough repetitive traction stress to lead to permanent stretching and drooping [11].

While young elite tennis players do not typically have tennis shoulder, they do have an observable alteration in the position of the scapula and the patterns of scapular motion in relation to the thoracic cage. This is known as scapular dyskinesia. In a study of 53 elite junior tennis players and 20 control study participants, 40 % of tennis players presented with scapular dyskinesia versus 10 % of control participants [101]. The malposition of the scapula leads to an increase of certain shoulder injuries. There are four different types of scapular dyskinesis. Type 1, inferomedial scapula border prominence, is associated with a tight anterior shoulder and weakness of the lower trapezius and serratus anterior. There is posterior tipping of the scapula that leads to a narrowed subacromial space. Type 2, medial border prominence, occurs due to trapezius and rhomboid fatigue. The medial border of the scapula is in a winged position at rest and is even more prominent in the cocking position.

Type 3, superomedial border prominence, has a high association with impingement and rotator cuff injury. In type 3 scapular dyskinesis, there are increased activation of the upper trapezius and miscommunication and discoordination between the upper and lower trapezius activity. This results in impingement due to loss of acromial elevation and posterior tilt [37]. Scapular dyskinesia has many etiologies including postural abnormality such as excessive lordosis or kyphosis or anatomical disruption including a history of a clavicle fracture or acromioclavicular joint injury [104]. Injury to certain nerves causes scapular dyskinesis from nerve palsy. Spinal accessory nerve (cranial nerve XI) deficit leads to trapezius weakness resulting in a depressed and laterally translated scapula. Long thoracic nerve (cervical nerves 5, 6, 7) injury leads to weakness of the serratus anterior causing superior and medial translation. Injury of the dorsal scapular nerve (cervical nerves 4, 5) causes scapular depression and lateral translation similar to spinal accessory nerve palsy [58]. Scapular dyskinesis is a broad term and does not suggest singular etiologies. It describes the loss of normal scapular control and motion. Other terms to describe this condition include 'floating scapula' and 'lateral scapula slide' [50]. Glenohumeral internal rotation deficit, described above, causes scapular dyskinesia. Scapular dyskinesia can also be caused by effusion or hemarthrosis. Increased pressure causes sensory receptors to obtain incorrect positional information. This proprioceptive deficit can deactivate neuromuscular pathways. While scapular dyskinesia has many etiologies, the abnormal control and motion cause common problems such as shoulder pain and impingement. The impingement is due to loss of protraction or retraction control. An increase in scapular protraction can lead to impingement of the supraspinatus and infraspinatus tendons, the superior joint capsule, the subacromial bursa, or the long head of the biceps brachii tendon. Overhead athletes typically have internal impingement, when the arm abducts and externally rotates which causes impingement between the posterosuperior labrum and the undersurface of the supraspinatus and infraspinatus tendons. The most common site for impingement is the supraspinatus tendon at the critical zone, which is its insertion site [26].

We recommend a physical therapy regimen with an experienced shoulder therapist for initial scapular dyskinesis treatment once a neurological etiology has been excluded. In general, during the acute injury phase (0–3 weeks), athletes are instructed not to abduct the arm greater than 90°. Patients must strengthen their hip and trunk by performing exercises such as abdominal crunches. Furthermore, they are encouraged to increase flexibility through trunk flexion/extension/rotation stretching. Increased trunk flexibility assists the scapula in protraction and retraction. The trunk is the focus initially because rehabilitation is based on a proximal to distal return of motion, control, and strength. During the acute phase, patients are also instructed to manually stretch their scalenes, levator scapulae, pectoralis minor, and posterior glenohumeral joint capsule.

Closed-chain kinetic exercises are begun before open-chain kinetic exercises because closed chain will help reinforce proprioceptive stimulation for joint mechanoreceptors. They also work by promoting muscle co-contraction which decreases shear force on the injured tissue [81]. During the recovery phase

(3–8 weeks), patients will progress to isometric, to active assistive, to concentric, and finally to eccentric muscular contractions. In the maintenance phase (6–10 weeks), patients will have achieved sufficient scapular control and motion. This phase focuses on plyometrics, combination open chain exercises, and sport-specific exercises [112].

Glenohumeral Joint Instability

Traumatic glenohumeral dislocations tend to occur in collision sports such as football and hockey. Approximately 98 % of these dislocations are anterior [39]. The incidence in tennis is unreported but can happen similarly to other sports after a fall or collision, not by an overhead racquet motion. 40 % of shoulder dislocations occur in patients under the age of 22 [15]; however, a shoulder dislocation in someone under the age of 10 is exceedingly rare. In the largest series of 500 patients, only 1.6 % occurred in patients under 10 years of age [96]. Recurrent dislocation and instability in patients less than 10 years of age approaches 100 % and in patients between 10 and 20 years of age are 94 % in athletes who return to sport and patients with open physes [1, 21, 72, 90, 92, 93, 96, 103]. This finding has led surgeons to recommend surgical stabilization following initial shoulder dislocations in young patients who are at a high risk for recurrence [1, 20, 80, 99].

As discussed above, true capsuloligamentous injury in the skeletally immature shoulder is rare. It has been suggested that the capsule of the pediatric shoulder is much more elastic than that of the adult's, allowing for more resilience [21, 86]. Furthermore, the insertion of the capsule on the glenoid is more laterally based in the skeletally immature patient, thereby resulting in a smaller anterior-inferior recess [94]. Once healed, this capsular anatomy would impart increased tension on the anterior capsule, suggesting that recurrent instability would be less likely [21]. Lastly, in the skeletally immature shoulder, the proximal humeral physis is extra-articular, except on the medial aspect of the physis, where the joint capsule attaches more distally along the humeral shaft. The capsular attachment to the epiphysis tends to fail first during dislocation, making physeal fractures possible after shoulder dislocation in skeletally immature patients. Because ligaments are up to seven times stronger than bone in young children, fractures are more common than ligamentous ruptures [59, 99]. Types of fracture include Salter-Harris type II epiphyseal separations in patients older than age 10 years and metaphyseal fractures in those younger than age 10 years [87]. Of those present with pure dislocations, Bankart lesions are not encountered in this population at the rate found in the young adult patient population [106]. Postacchini et al. reported 33 patients aged 12–17 years with anterior dislocation and found only 1 Bankart lesion in the 7 patients less than 14 years [86]. Cordischi et al. found no Bankart lesions in 14 skeletally immature patients who sustained an anterior dislocation [17]. Conversely, in patients aged 17–23 years, 97 % had a Bankart lesion and 91 % had a Hill-Sachs lesion [106].

Traumatic shoulder instability presents with obvious deformity, pain, and limitations in shoulder range of motion. In a true dislocation (as opposed to a subluxation), the arm is typically adducted and internally rotated in an anteroinferior dislocation. Upon presentation, a thorough neurovascular examination should be performed. The axillary nerve is the most commonly injured neurovascular structure and rates of injury have been reported up to 42 % [111]. A full shoulder dislocation radiographic series with orthogonal views should be obtained: AP, Grashey, scapula Y view, axillary, and Stryker notch view. The proximal humeral physis should be evaluated closely because it can be injured at the time of dislocation and/or during reduction. An MRI is rarely necessary, nor practical, in the acute setting. However, it does provide details regarding the concomitant soft-tissue injuries after a shoulder dislocation. The status of the labral tissue and presence of a bony or soft-tissue Bankart lesion may affect treatment decisions of the skeletally immature patient with a shoulder dislocation.

Following reduction the management hinges on the age of the patient. For patients older than 14 years or with closed physis, they should be managed as adult patients with glenohumeral joint instability. With regard to those younger than 14 years, it depends on whether they are a first-time or recurrent dislocator. First-time dislocators can be managed with rehabilitation and nonsurgical treatment. In recurrent dislocators, an MRI arthrogram should be obtained. In those patients with a Bankart lesion on MR, surgical stabilization is indicated. Those without a Bankart lesion can be treated as a first-time dislocator [65].

Atraumatic multidirectional instability is more common in the young athlete and usually occurs due to recurrent microtrauma or in association with generalized ligamentous laxity. In the overhead motion, the tennis player with recurrent instability often complains of pain during late cocking and early acceleration phases. They often complain of decreased performance with diminished velocity and/or loss of control. Examination in this setting must include an assessment of load shift testing for glenohumeral translation, presence of a sulcus sign, apprehension and relocation testing, and an evaluation for generalized ligamentous laxity. As in acute instability, an instability radiographic series should be obtained. MRI may help assess soft tissue disruption such as a Bankart lesion. Treatment for macroinstability in the young tennis player follows an algorithm similar to that for instability in a mature throwing athlete. The only exception is that nonoperative management should be attempted for a longer period of time in the young athlete. Surgery in the patient with habitual voluntary multidirectional instability is fraught with complications and recurrences [34, 95] and should be avoided unless left with no choice. In those patients who fail nonoperative treatment, surgical reconstruction can be considered with an arthroscopic capsular imbrication procedure. It is of critical importance to understand the extent and direction of instability beforehand so that the appropriate tissues are tightened. Any reconstruction must recognize the need to minimize loss of external rotation in the tennis player, which can negatively impact their serve and stroke.

Microinstabilty with complaints of pain and diminished performance is much more commonly seen in overhead athletes than macroinstability [39, 40, 55, 77, 83]. In these athletes, instability is not the primary presenting symptom. On physical examination, the athlete will demonstrate findings consistent with rotator cuff inflammation with positive impingement signs and supraspinatus weakness. These are not primary findings, but rather secondary to underlying instability. Subtle asymmetry of glenohumeral translation and differences in apprehension and relocation tests between the affected and unaffected sides are critical to diagnosis. Routine radiographs are almost always normal. Treatment is initially nonoperative with an emphasis on symptomatic management with rest, avoidance of tennis, and anti-inflammatory medications. Once asymptomatic, a dynamic stabilization program of rotator cuff and periscapular strengthening can be initiated. Surgical treatment with anterior stabilization is rarely necessary.

Little Leaguer's Shoulder

Little leaguer's shoulder has also gone by the names proximal humeral epiphysiolysis and slipped capital humeral epiphysis. It was initially described by Dotter in 1953 [22]. Little leaguer's shoulder is unique to overhead sports athletes with open growth plates. It is thought to be an overuse or stress injury of the proximal humeral physis that occurs secondary to shear and distraction caused by rotational forces about the shoulder [82]. The average age of onset is 14 years and these patients typically present with lateral shoulder pain during overhead activities. Most patients report insidious onset of symptoms that have been present for months and often delay seeking consultation until the pain increases or there is diminishment in overhead velocity or control [82].

Up to 70 % of patients with little leaguer's shoulder have tenderness over the proximal and lateral portion of the humeral head. Radiographs should be ordered to confirm the diagnosis: anteroposterior in internal and external rotation, lateral Y-view and axillary views, and comparison views of the uninvolved side. Classic findings include widening of the proximal humeral physis with or without physeal fragmentation, sclerosis, and demineralization (Fig. 8.5) [13, 82]. Severe slippage is not usually present. If radiographs are negative, but the condition is suspected, an MRI can be obtained. In the early phases, prior to separation, an MRI will show significant edema around the physis (Fig. 8.6).

Treatment consists of relative rest from tennis, icing, and analgesic medications as needed for pain [13]. The athlete should be placed on complete rest of the shoulder for at least 3 weeks [11]. Range of motion activities can begin after 3 weeks, followed by strengthening exercises at 8 weeks if the patient is asymptomatic. Athletes are encouraged to maintain cardiovascular conditioning. Patients should begin a groundstroke program when they are pain-free and have rested from tennis for at least 4–6 months [11]. Other authors recommend delaying practicing sport-specific skills for as long as 1 year [29]. We will typically get an MRI if this condition is suspected and not obvious on radiograph. A follow-up MRI may be obtained to ensure resolution of the bone edema that typically occurs. Evaluation of serving and groundstroke mechanics should also be considered as well as the frequency and duration of practices.

Since the proximal humerus has great growth potential in children under 12 years of age, slips of up to 50 % or 40° of angulation can often be remodeled and surgery is not necessary [61].

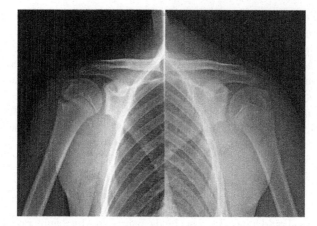

Fig. 8.5 Radiographs demonstrating the classic findings of widening of the proximal humeral physis (*left*) compared to the normal contralateral side (*right*) in little leaguer's shoulder

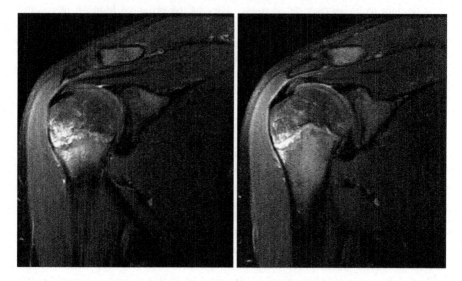

Fig. 8.6 Magnetic resonance imaging of little leaguer's shoulder demonstrating significant edema around the physis

Proximal Humerus Fractures

Acute fractures of the proximal humerus account for less than 5 % of all pediatric fractures [16, 18, 19, 30]. These fractures preferentially involve the physis and have a peak incidence at age 15 years [19]. Most fractures are Salter-Harris II injuries that result from rapid growth and resultant weakness of the physis [8]. This is a dramatic injury that occurs with a single serve. Prodromal arm pain may or may not have been present. The athlete commonly has acute pain that is exacerbated by any movement of the arm. Plain radiographs are diagnostic. Because severe displacement is uncommon, treatment is routinely nonoperative. However, in the case of significant displacement, surgical treatment is required, especially if the athlete is close to skeletal maturity with little time for fracture remodeling [16, 42]. Options for fixation include closed reduction with percutaneous pinning.

Acromioclavicular Joint Separation

A sprain of the acromioclavicular (AC) joint usually occurs as a result of a blow to the top of the shoulder. Rockwood has developed a classification of AC injuries that is widely used [94]. We recommend obtaining bilateral Zanca views on a single cassette. We have found this to be the most reliable way to visualize the acromioclavicular joints and grade the injury. In addition, we always obtain an axillary view (essential for diagnosing a type IV injury). In a type I injury, there is complete congruity of the distal clavicle and acromion. In the type II injury, there is incomplete overlap of the clavicle and acromion. In the type III injury, the clavicle and acromion are completely separated, as a result of complete rupture of the AC and coracoclavicular ligaments. Types IV, V, and VI are variations of the completely disrupted AC joint, with the clavicle being displaced posteriorly, superiorly, or inferiorly, respectively.

Type I and II AC joint sprains may be treated nonoperatively in a sling until the patient can tolerate carrying the arm freely (days to weeks). As soon as possible, the patient should begin pendulum exercises and advance to exercises to strengthen the trapezius and deltoid muscles. Athletes with type I sprains can usually return to activity in 7–10 days, whereas type II sprains usually require an additional 4 weeks [28].

In type III and V injuries, tenting of the skin may be present. In such a case, operative treatment is mandatory to maintain skin integrity. Otherwise, the management of type III injuries remains controversial. Both nonoperative and operative treatments have been described, with some authors advocating surgery for type III in young, active patients [31, 63, 68, 97]. We believe that because tennis players place such high functional demands on the acromioclavicular joint, type III injuries should be operatively fixed.

Unlike type III injuries, there is no controversy regarding surgical treatment in type IV, V, and VI injuries. Type VI injuries are extremely rare. We prefer to use a modified Mazzocca reconstruction of the coracoclavicular ligaments [12] for operative treatment of type III, IV, V, and VI AC joint separations.

Distal Clavicle Osteolysis

Osteolysis of the distal clavicle is an overuse injury from repetitive microtrauma. It has also been described as a sequelae following a traumatic injury to the distal clavicle or acromioclavicular joint (type I or II separations) [98]. While the most common presentation is in adult weightlifters, this entity has been also identified in young athletes who are weight training year-round for high-level sports [53, 55]. Patients present with subtle complaints of acromioclavicular pain after workouts; this eventually progresses to interfere with training and activities of daily living. On examination, there is tenderness to palpation of the distal clavicle at the AC joint and pain with cross-body adduction. Treatment primarily consists of rest and anti-inflammatory medications; a cortisone injection to reduce the capsular inflammation can be considered. For those who fail nonoperative treatment, distal clavicle resection usually results in resolution of pain and return to sport [98]. We perform an isolated distal clavicle resection as described by Flatow et al. [27] from a superior approach in athletes that have no other shoulder pathology. Long-term follow-up has demonstrated excellent outcomes and comparable results to an open approach [121].

Clavicle Fractures

Clavicle fractures are among the most common fractures in childhood. They account for 10–15 % of all childhood fracture [6]. The typical mechanism of injury is a fall on the point of the shoulder. More than 80 % of clavicle fractures occur in the middle third. Prognosis for these fractures is excellent given the significant growth potential of the bone. For middle third fractures which are not significantly displaced, the arm should be placed in a sling. The sling should be used during waking hours for at least the first 2 weeks or until the patient can carry the arm without discomfort [28]. Surgical treatment is indicated in open fractures, neurovascular compromise, and gross displacement with skin at risk for perforation [57]. Injuries to the sternoclavicular and acromioclavicular joints in a pediatric patient are physeal injuries until proven otherwise. The medial clavicle physis is the last physis to close at 22–25 years of age. Ligaments attached to thick periosteum are significantly stronger than the physis, resulting in physeal fracture more commonly than dislocation. Because of the remodeling potential, excellent results are achieved for medial and lateral physeal fractures with a sling and symptomatic treatment [6].

The management of clavicle fractures in patients 15–20 years of age is controversial [118]. Despite open physes, these patients have less growth remaining and decreased remodeling potential. Clear indications for operative intervention still remain the same: compromised skin or a neurovascular deficit. A relative indication is a displaced or Z-type fracture with an intercalary comminuted segment. In 2013 the Cochrane Group published a systematic review examining surgical versus conservative treatment of middle third clavicle fractures [64]. Eight trials were included and no statistical difference in outcomes was found. However, one must keep in mind that all of the randomized trials concerning clavicle fractures to date have reported a 15–20 % nonunion rate with nonoperative treatment and that malunions are common, contrary to consistent union and low rates of complication in operative treatment [74, 91]. It is clear that some patients benefit from operative fixation, but hard indications for fracture fixation are lacking in the literature. It is reasonable, however, to consider

shortening, comminution, acute scapular winging as a result of distal fragment translation, and concomitant polytrauma as relative indications for surgery [60, 89, 116].
Due to the importance of the clavicle in transferring forces from the core to the shoulder in tennis, gross angulation or shortening of the clavicle should be considered
when determining which treatment would best suit the athlete.

Long-Term Sequelae of Tennis

Due to the high incidence of shoulder pathology in tennis players, some have ques-
tioned whether those participating in tennis are at increased risk of primary glenohumeral arthritis as they age. One investigation studied 18 senior tennis players with
no history of shoulder surgery or trauma and compared them to age-matched controls using radiographs [71]. Results showed that 33 % of the tennis players had
radiographic signs of degenerative changes in the glenohumeral joint of their dominant arm versus only 11 % of matched controls.

Conclusion

The popularity of tennis shows no signs of dwindling and young athletes must begin
training at an early age to play at the elite level. Shoulder injuries are common in this
demographic as a result of the high stresses tennis places on the shoulder suspensory
complex (SSC). In the elite youth players, there has been an increase in playing time,
throughout the year with no downtime, and less time for participation in other sports.
This places increased stress on the shoulder with more risk of developing overuse
injuries. By understanding the pathology, the normal development, and the biomechanical demands of the sport, healthcare providers can treat athletes more efficiently,
allowing for faster and safer returns to tennis after injury. In young players, we advocate for early identification of poor technique, physical deficits, and injury patterns so
that nonoperative rehabilitation can prevent progressive worsening and more serious
or chronic injury. It is clear that young tennis athletes are at risk for developing shoulder pathology and the surgeon, physician, athletic trainer, physical therapist, and
coach need to keep this fact at the forefront as they care for these players.

References

1. Arciero RA, Wheeler JH, Ryan JB, McBride JT. Arthroscopic Bankart repair versus nonoperative treatment for acute, initial anterior shoulder dislocations. Am J Sports Med.
   1994;22(5):589–94.
2. Bach HG, Goldberg BA. Posterior capsular contracture of the shoulder. J Am Acad Orthop
   Surg. 2006;14:265–77.

3. Baxter-Jones A, Maffulli N, Helms P. Low injury rates in elite athletes. Arch Dis Child. 1993;68:130–2.
4. Beachy G, Akau CK, Martinson M, et al. High school sports injuries. A longitudinal study at Punahou School: 1988 to 1996. Am J Sports Med. 1997;25:675–81.
5. Benjamin HJ, Briner Jr WW. Little league elbow. Clin J Sport Med. 2005;15:37–40.
6. Bishop JY, Flatow EL. Paediatric shoulder trauma. Clin Orthop Relat Res. 2005 Mar;(432):41–8.
7. Brenner D, Elliston C, Hall E, et al. Estimated risks of radiation-induced fatal cancer from pediatric CT. AJR Am J Roentgenol. 2001;176(2):289–96.
8. Bright RW, Burstein AH, Elmore SM. Epiphyseal-plate cartilage. A biomechanical and histological analysis of failure modes. J Bone Joint Surg. 1974;56A:688–703.
9. Burkhart SS, Morgan CD. The peel-back mechanism: its role in producing and extending posterior type II SLAP lesions and its effect on SLAP repair rehabilitation. Arthroscopy. 1998;14:637–40.
10. Burkhart SS, Morgan CD, Kibler WB. Shoulder injuries in overhead athletes: the "dead arm" revisited. Clin Sports Med. 2000;19:125–58.
11. Bylak J, Hutchinson MR. Common sports injuries in young tennis players. Sport Med 1998;26:119–32.
12. Carofino BC, Mazzocca AD. The anatomic coracoclavicular ligament reconstruction: surgical technique and indications. J Shoulder Elbow Surg. 2010;19(2 Suppl):37–46.
13. Carson Jr WG, Gasser SI. Little Leaguer's shoulder. A report of 23 cases. Am J Sports Med. 1998;26:575–80.
14. Chandler TJ, Kibler WB, Stragener EC. Shoulder strength, power, and endurance in college tennis players. Am J Sports Med. 1992;20(4):455–8.
15. Cleeman E, Flatow EL. Shoulder dislocations in the young patient. Orthop Clin North Am. 2000;31(2):217–29.
16. Cohn BT, Froimson AL. Salter 3 fracture dislocation of glenohumeral joint in a 10-year-old. Orthop Rev. 1986;15:403–4.
17. Cordischi K, Li X, Busconi B. Immediate outcomes after primary traumatic anterior shoulder dislocation in skeletally immature patients aged 10 to 13 years. Orthopedics. 2009;32(9):1.
18. Curtis RJJ, Dameron Jr TB, Rockwood Jr CA. Fractures and dislocations of the shoulder in children. In: Rockwood CAJ, Wilkins KE, King RE, editors. Fractures in children. Philadelphia: JB Lippincott; 1991. p. 829–919.
19. Dameron Jr TB, Riebel DB. Fracture involving the proximal humeral epiphyseal plate. J Bone Joint Surg. 1969;51A:289–97.
20. DeBerardino TM, Arciero RA, Taylor DC, Uhorchak JM. Prospective evaluation of arthroscopic stabilization of acute, initial anterior shoulder dislocations in young athletes: Two-to-five-year follow-up. Am J Sports Med. 2001;29(5):586–92.
21. Deitch J, Mehlman CT, Foad SL, et al. Traumatic anterior shoulder dislocation in adolescents. Am J Sports Med. 2003;31(5):758–63.
22. Dotter WB. Little leaguer's shoulder: a fracture of the proximal epiphyseal cartilage of the humerus due to baseball pitching. Guthrie Clin Bull. 1953;23:58.
23. Elliot B. Biomechanics and tennis. Br J Sports Med. 2006;40(5):392–6.
24. Elliott B, Fleisig G, Nicholls R, Escamilla R. Technique effects on upper limb loading in the tennis serve. J Sci Med Sport. 2003;6(1):76–87.
25. Elliott B, Reid M, Crespo M, editors. Biomechanics of advanced tennis. London: International Tennis Federation; 2003. p. 33–47.
26. Escamilla RF, Hooks TR, Wilk KE. Optimal management of shoulder impingement syndrome. J Sports Med. 2014;5:13–24.
27. Flatow EL, Duralde XA, Nicholson GP, Pollock RG, Bigliani LU. Arthroscopic resection of the distal clavicle with a superior approach. J Shoulder Elbow Surg. 1995;4(1 Pt 1):41–50.
28. Gomez JE. Upper extremity injuries in youth sports. Pediatr Clin North Am. 2002;49:593–626.

29. Gregg JR, Torg E. Upper extremity injuries in adolescent tennis players. Clin Sports Med. 1988;7(2):371–85.
30. Gregg-Smith SJ, White SH. Salter-Harris III fracture-dislocation of the proximal humeral epiphysis. Injury. 1992;23:199–200.
31. Gstettner C, Tauber M, Hitzl W, Resch H. Rockwood type III acromioclavicular dislocation: surgical versus conservative treatment. J Shoulder Elbow Surg. 2008;17(2):220–5.
32. Hanchard NC, Lenza M, Handoll HH, Takwoingi Y. Physical tests for shoulder impingements and local lesions of bursa, tendon or labrum that may accompany impingement. Cochrane Database Syst Rev. 2013;4:CD007427.
33. Hennig EM. Influence of racket properties on injuries and performance in tennis. Exerc Sport Sci Rev. 2007;35:62–6.
34. Huber H, Gerber C. Voluntary subluxation of the shoulder in children. A long-term follow-up study of 36 shoulders. J Bone Joint Surg. 1994;76B:118–22.
35. Hutchinson MR, Laprade RF, Burnett 2nd QM, et al. Injury surveillance at the UTSA Boys' Tennis Championships: a 6-year study. Med Sci Sports Exerc. 1995;27:826–30.
36. Hyman M. Young athletes, big league pain. Business Week. 7 June 2004.
37. Iannoti J, et al. Disorders of the shoulder diagnosis and management: shoulder reconstruction. LWW;Philadelphia, PA. 3rd ed. 2014. p. 597.
38. Ide J, Maeda S, Takagi K. Sports activity after arthroscopic superior labral repair using suture anchors in overhead-throwing athletes. Am J Sports Med. 2005;33:507–14.
39. Ireland ML, Andrews JR. Shoulder and elbow injuries in the young athlete. Clin Sports Med. 1988;7:473–94.
40. Ireland ML, Satterwhite YE. Shoulder injuries. In: Andrews JR, Zarins B, Wilk KE, editors. Injuries in baseball. Philadelphia: Lippincott-Raven; 1998. p. 271–81.
41. Itoi E, et al. Tensile properties of the supraspinatus tendon. J Orthop Res. 1995;13(4):578–84.
42. Jaberg H, Warner JJ, Jakob RP. Percutaneous stabilization of unstable fractures of the humerus. J Bone Joint Surg Am. 1992;74:508–15.
43. Jayanthi N, Sallay PI, Hunker P, et al. Skill-level related injuries in recreational competition tennis players. Med Sci Tennis. 2005;10:12–5.
44. Jobe FW, Motnes DR, Tibone JE. An EMG analysis of shoulder in pitching: a second report. Am J Sports Med. 1984;12:218–20.
45. Jobe FW. An EMG, analysis of the shoulder in throwing and pitching, a preliminary report. Am J Sports Med. 1983;11:3–5.
46. Plancher KD, Litchfield R, Hawkins RJ. Rehabilitation of the shoulder in tennis players. Clin Sports Med. 1995;14:111–37.
47. Kibler W, Chandler J. Racquet sports. In: Fu FH, Sone DA, editors. Sports injuries – mechanism, prevention, and treatment. Baltimore: Williams & Wilkins; 1994. p. 278–92.
48. Kibler WB, Chandler TJ, Uhl TL, et al. A musculoskeletal approach to the preparticipation physical examination: preventing injury and improving performance. Am J Sports Med. 1989;17:525–31.
49. Kibler WB, Chandler TJ. Musculoskeletal adaptations and injuries associated with intense participation in youth sports. In: Cahill BR, Pearl AJ, editors. Intensive participation in children's sports. Park Ridge: American Academy of Orthopedic Surgeons; 1993. p. 2–7.
50. Kibler WB, Chandler TJ. Range of motion in junior tennis players participating in an injury risk modification program. J Sci Med Sport. 2003;6:51–62.
51. Kibler WB, McQueen C, Uhl TL. Fitness evaluations and fitness findings in competitive junior tennis players. Clin Sports Med. 1988;7:403–16.
52. Kibler WB. The role of the scapula in throwing motion. Contemp Orthop. 1991;22:525–32.
53. Kim HK, Crotty E. Post-traumatic osteolysis of the distal clavicle. Pediatr Radiol. 2010;40:784.
54. Kim SH, Ha KI, Kim SH, Choi HJ. Results of arthroscopic treatment of superior labral lesions. J Bone Joint Surg Am. 2002;84:981–5.

55. Kocher MS, Waters PM, Micheli LJ. Upper extremity injuries in the paediatric athlete. Sports Med. 2000;2:117–35.
56. Kovacs M, Ellenbecker T. An 8-stage model for evaluating the tennis serve: implications for performance enhancement and injury prevention. Sports Health. 2011;3(6):504–13.
57. Kubiak R, Slongo T. Operative treatment of clavicle fractures in children: a review of 21 year. J Pediatr Orthop. 2002;22:736–9.
58. Kuhn JE, Plancher KD, Hawkins RJ. Scapular winging. J Am Acad Orthop Surg. 1995;3:319–25.
59. Lampert C, Baumgartner G, Slongo T, Kohler G, Horst M. Traumatic shoulder dislocation in children and adolescents: a multicenter retrospective analysis. Eur J Trauma. 2002;29(6):375–8.
60. Ledger M, Leeks N, Ackland T, Wang A. Short malunions of the clavicle: an anatomic and functional study. J Shoulder Elbow Surg. 2005;14:349–54.
61. Lefèvre Y, Journeau P, Angelliaume A, Bouty A, Dobremez E. Proximal humerus fractures in children and adolescents. Orthop Traumatol Surg Res. 2014;100(1 Suppl):S149–56.
62. Lehman RC. Shoulder pain in the competitive tennis player. Clin Sports Med. 1988;7:309–27.
63. Leidel BA, Braunstein V, Kirschhoff C, Pilotto S, Mutschler W, Biberthaler P. Consistency of long-term outcome of acute Rockwood acromioclavicular joint separations after K-wire transfixation. J Trauma. 2009;66(6):1666–71.
64. Lenza M, Buchbinder R, Johnston RV, Belloti JC, Faloppa F. Surgical versus conservative interventions for treating fractures of the middle third of the clavicle. Cochrane Database Syst Rev. 2013;6(6).
65. Li X, Ma R, Nielsen N, Gulotta LV, Dines JS, Owens BD. Management of shoulder instability in the skeletally immature patient. J Am Acad Orthop Surg. 2013;21:529–37.
66. Lieberman J. AAOS comprehensive review. American Academy of Orthopaedic Surgeons; Rosemont, Illinois: Vol. 2. Section 8. 2009. p. 793–804.
67. Lintner D, Mayol M, Uzodinma O, Jones R, Labossiere D. Glenohumeral internal rotation deficits in professional pitchers enrolled in an internal rotation stretching program. Am J Sports Med. 2007;35:617–21.
68. Lizaur A, Sanz-Reig J, Gonzalez-Parreno S. Long-term results of the surgical treatment of type III acromioclavicular dislocations: an update of a previous report. J Bone Joint Surg Br. 2011;93(8):1088–92.
69. Maenhout A, et al. Quantifying acromiohumeral distance in overhead athletes with glenohumeral internal rotation loss and the influence of a stretching program. Am J Sports Med. 2012;40(9):2105–12.
70. Manske RC, Grant-Nierman M, Lucas B. Shoulder posterior internal impingement in the overhead athlete. Int J Sports Phys Ther. 2013;8(2):194–204.
71. Maquirriain J, Ghisi JP, Amato S. Is tennis a predisposing factor for degenerative shoulder disease? A controlled study in former elite players. Br J Sports Med. 2006;40:447–50.
72. Marans HJ, Angel KR, Schemitsch EH, et al. The fate of traumatic anterior dislocation of the shoulder in children. J Bone Joint Surg Am. 1992;74(8):1242–4.
73. McCann PD, Bigliani LU. Shoulder pain in tennis players. Sports Med. 1994;17(1):53–64.
74. McKee RC, Whelan DB, Schemitsch EH, McKee MD. Operative versus no care of displaced midshaft clavicular fractures: a meta-analysis of randomized clinical trials. J Bone Joint Surg Am. 2012;94:675–84.
75. Neuman BJ, Boisvert CB, Reiter B, Lawson K, Ciccotti MG, Cohen SB. Results of arthroscopic repair of type II superior labral anterior posterior lesions in overhead athletes: assessment of return to preinjury playing level and satisfaction. Am J Sports Med. 2011;39(9):1883–8.
76. Nirschl RP. Rotator cuff tendinitis: basic concepts of pathoetiology. In: Barr JS, editor. Instructional course lectures 38. Park Ridge: American Academy of Orthopedic Surgeons; 1989. p. 439–45.
77. Oberlander MA, Chisar MA, Campbell B. Epidemiology of shoulder injuries in throwing and overhead athletes. Sports Med Arthrosc Rev. 2000;8:115–23.

78. Ogden JA. Radiologic aspects. In: Ogden JA, editor. Skeletal injury in the child. Philadelphia: WB Saunders; 1990. p. 65–96.
79. Owens BD, Goss TP. The floating shoulder. J Bone Joint Surg Br. 2006;88-B:1419–24.
80. Owens BD, DeBerardino TM, Nelson BJ, et al. Long-term follow-up of acute arthroscopic Bankart repair for initial anterior shoulder dislocations in young athletes. Am J Sports Med. 2009;37(4):669–73.
81. Palmer LM, Epler ME. Fundamentals of musculoskeletal assessment techniques. 2nd ed. Lippincott: Williams & Wilkins; 1998. p. 106–24.
82. Patel DR, Nelson TL. Sports injuries in adolescents. Med Clin North Am. 2000;84:983–1007.
83. Patel PR, Warner JJP. Shoulder injuries in the skeletally immature athlete. Sports Med Arthrosc Rev. 1996;4:99–113.
84. Pluim BM, Staal JB, Windler GE, et al. Tennis injuries: occurrence, aetiology, and prevention. Br J Sports Med. 2006;40:415–23.
85. Pluim BM, Staal JB. Tennis. In: Caine DJ, Harmer P, Schiff M, editors. Epidemiology of injury in Olympic sports. Oxford: Wiley Blackwell; 2010. p. 277–93.
86. Postacchini F, Gumina S, Cinotti G. Anterior shoulder dislocation in adolescents. J Shoulder Elbow Surg. 2000;9(6):470–4.
87. Price CT, Flynn JM. Management of fractures. In: Lovell WW, Winter RB, Morrissy RT, Weinstein SL, editors. Lovell and Winter's pediatric orthopaedics. Philadelphia: Lippincott Williams and Wilkins; 2005. p. 1430–528.
88. Priest JD, Nagel DA. Tennis shoulder. Am J Sports Med. 1976;4:28–42.
89. Ristevski B, Hall JA, Pearce D, Potter J, Farrugia M, McKee MD. The radiographic quantification of scapular malalignment after malunion of displaced clavicular shaft fractures. J Shoulder Elbow Surg. 2013;22:240–6.
90. Robinson CM, Dobson RJ. Anterior instability of the shoulder after trauma. J Bone Joint Surg Br. 2004;86(4):469–79.
91. Robinson CM, Goudie EB, Murray IR, Jenkins PJ, Ahktar MA, Read EO, Foster CJ, Clark K, Brooksbank AJ, Arthur A, Crowther MA, Packham I, Cheeser TJ. Open reduction and plate fixation versus nonoperative treatment for displaced midshaft clavicular fractures: a multicenter, randomized, controlled trial. J Bone Joint Surg Am. 2013;95:1576–84.
92. Robinson CM, Howes J, Murdoch H, Will E, Graham C. Functional outcome and risk of recurrent instability after primary traumatic anterior shoulder dislocation in young patients. J Bone Joint Surg Am. 2006;88(11):2326–36.
93. Robinson CM, Kelly M, Wakefield AE. Redislocation of the shoulder during the first six weeks after a primary anterior dislocation: risk factors and results of treatment. J Bone Joint Surg Am. 2002;84(9):1552–9.
94. Rockwood C, Matsen F. The shoulder. Philadelphia: WB Saunders; 1990.
95. Rowe CR, Pierce DS, Clark JG. Voluntary dislocation of the shoulder: a preliminary report on a clinical, electromyographic and psychiatric study of twenty-six patients. J Bone Joint Surg. 1973;55A:445–60.
96. Rowe CR. Prognosis in dislocations of the shoulder. J Bone Joint Surg Am. 1956;38-A(5):957–77.
97. Ryhanen J, Niemela E, Kaarela O, Raatikainen T. Stabilization of acute, complete acromioclavicular joint dislocations with a new C hook implant. J Shoulder Elbow Surg. 2003;12(5):442–5.
98. Schwarzkopf R, Ishak C, Elman M, Gelber J, Strauss DN, Jazrawi LM. Distal clavicular osteolysis: a review of the literature. Bull NYU Hosp Jt Dis. 2008;66(2):94–101.
99. Seybold D, Schildhauer TA, Muhr G. Rare anterior shoulder dislocation in a toddler. Arch Orthop Trauma Surg. 2009;129(3):295–8.
100. Shepard MF, Dugas JR, Zeng N, Andrews JR. Differences in the ultimate strength of the biceps anchor and the generation of the type II superior labral anterior posterior lesions in a cadaveric model. Am J Sports Med. 2004;32(5):1197–201.
101. Silva R, et al. Clinical and ultrasonographic correlation between scapular dyskinesia and subacromial space measurement among junior elite tennis players. Br J Sports Med. 2010;44:407–10.

102. Silva RT, Takahashi R, Berra B, et al. Medical assistance at the Brazilian juniors tennis circuit – a one-year prospective study. J Sci Med Sport. 2003;6:14–8.
103. Simonet WT, Cofield RH. Prognosis in anterior shoulder dislocation. Am J Sports Med. 1984;12(1):19–24.
104. Smith R, et al. Anatomical characteristics of the upper serratus anterior: cadaver dissection. J Orthop Sports Phys Ther. 2003;33:449–53.
105. Snyder SJ, Karzel RP, Del Pizzo W, et al. SLAP lesions of the shoulder. Arthroscopy. 1990;6:274–9.
106. Taylor DC, Arciero RA. Pathologic changes associated with shoulder dislocations: arthroscopic and physical examination findings in first-time, traumatic anterior dislocations. Am J Sports Med. 1997;25(3):306–11.
107. Torres RR, Gomes JL. Measurement of glenohumeral internal rotation in asymptomatic tennis players and swimmers. Am J Sports Med. 2009;37(5):1017–23.
108. Tsur A, Gillson S. Brachial biceps tendon injuries in young female high-level tennis players. Croat Med J. 2000;41:184–5.
109. Tyler TF, et al. Correction of posterior shoulder tightness is associated with symptom resolution in patients with internal impingement. Am J Sports Med. 2010;38(1):114–9.
110. Tyler TF, Nicholas SJ, Roy T, Gleim GW. Quantification of posterior capsule tightness and motion loss in patients with shoulder impingement. Am J Sports Med. 2000;28:668–73.
111. Visser CP, Coene LN, Brand R, Tavy DL. the incidence of nerve injury in anterior dislocation of the shoulder and its influences on functional recovery: a prospective clinical and EMG study. J Bone Joint Surg Br. 1999;81(4):679–85.
112. Voight ML, Thomson BC. The role of the scapula in the rehabilitation of shoulder injuries. J Athl Train. 2000;35(3):364–72.
113. Warner JD, Micheli LJ, Arlanian LE, et al. Patterns of flexibility, laxity, and strength in normal shoulders and shoulders with instability and impingement. Am J Sports Med. 1990;18:366–75.
114. Wei SH, Chiang JY, Shiang TY, et al. Comparison of shock transmission and forearm electromyography between experienced and recreational tennis players during backhand strokes. Clin J Sport Med. 2006;16:129–35.
115. Weiss JM, Arkader A, Wells LM, Ganley TJ. Rotator cuff injuries in adolescent athletes. J Pediatr Orthop B. 2013;22:133–7.
116. Wick M, Muller EJ, Kollig E, Muhr G. Midshaft fractures of the clavicle with a shortening of more than 2 cm predispose to nonunion. Arch Orthop Trauma Surg. 2001;121:207–11.
117. Winge S, Jørgensen U, Lassen Nielsen A. Epidemiology of injuries in Danish championship tennis. Int J Sports Med. 1989;10:368–71.
118. Yang S, Werner BC, Gwathmey Jr FW. Treatment trends in adolescent clavicle fractures. J Pediatr Orhtop. 2015;35(3):229–33.
119. Yoneda M. Arthroscopic capsular release for painful throwing shoulder with posterior capsular tightness. Arthroscopy. 2006;22(7):801.e1–5.
120. Zattara M, Bouisset S. Posturo-kinetic organization during the early phase of voluntary upper limb movement. J Neurol Neurosurg Psychiatry. 1988;5:956–65.
121. Zawadsky M, Marra G, Wiater JM, Levine WN, Pollock RG, Flatow EL, Bigliani LU. Osteolysis of the distal clavicle: long-term results of arthroscopic resection. Arthroscopy. 2000;16(6):600–5.

Chapter 9
Elbow, Wrist, and Hand Injuries in the Young Tennis Athlete

Steve Wang and Michael Hausman

Tennis is a global sport, with tens of millions of yearly participants worldwide and over 200 nations having an association with the International Tennis Federation. Tennis carries with it a unique profile of upper extremity injuries. The equipment, biomechanics, and physical demands result in an injury profile that can cause varying degrees of disability and possible absence from school. This can have substantial consequences on the young athlete on a personal and a societal level. Knowledge of the spectrum of injuries and its risk factors are important to discover the potential for prevention, treatment, and speedy recovery of our young players.

Who Gets Injured?

The increasing competitive nature of tennis places the growing athlete at great demands. Children with promising talent are identified, tracked, coached, and developed at younger ages, and their musculoskeletal systems are immature and vulnerable to injuries not common in adult professional athletes. Ossification is incomplete, and cartilage and ligaments cannot withstand repeated supraphysiologic loading without potential deformation and damage. Concurrently, the level of competition increases the demand for a faster serve and more playing time. The majority of injuries associated with tennis playing are due to force overload of the muscle-tendon-bone unit, rather than acute trauma [1]. In high-level players under 18 years of age, injury rates have been estimated to be anywhere from 2 to 20

S. Wang
Kaiser Permanente Moanalua Medical Center, Hawaii, USA

M. Hausman, (✉)
Department of Orthopaedic Surgery, Mount Sinai Medical Center, New York, NY, USA
e-mail: Michael.Hausman@mountsinai.org

© Springer International Publishing Switzerland 2016   167
A.C. Colvin, J.N. Gladstone (eds.), *The Young Tennis Player: Injury Prevention and Treatment*, Contemporary Pediatric and Adolescent Sports Medicine,
DOI 10.1007/978-3-319-27559-8_9

injuries per 1000 h of tennis played [2–4]. Such findings are consistent with use-related injury patterns found in skeletally immature baseball players, where strict throwing limits and pitch counts have been recommended.

More female athletes are playing tennis. Females have been reported to have lower average upper body strength compared to their male counterparts, leading to more upper extremity injuries [1]. Expectations of a higher injury prevalence among female competitors would be expected; however, epidemiological studies show an equal rate of upper extremity injuries across genders [5].

What Are the Risk Factors?

The active playing time has been correlated with injury rates, such as tennis elbow [6]. Although there is data that an athlete's skill level has not made a difference in injury rates [7], there have been studies to show that less experienced players subject themselves to higher stresses when playing. These studies correlated a lower skill level with higher vibrations at the wrist and elbow during the backhand stroke [8, 9]. The authors theorized that the more novice players may use a higher grip force, leading to higher vibrations and an increased chance of injury. It is possible that the experienced player, generating power with a fully developed, well-integrated stroke, may have decreased damaging forces, but their increased volume of play puts them at a similar risk of injury as the more novice player [10].

Racket grip position has also been studied and associated with certain types of injuries. Tagliafico found that ulnar-sided injuries (extensor carpi ulnaris tendonitis and triangular fibrocartilage complex pathology) were significantly associated with Western or semi-Western grips, while radial-sided injuries (flexor carpi radialis tendonitis, deQuervain's tendinopathy, and intersection syndrome) were more commonly found in players with the Eastern grip [11] (Fig. 9.1).

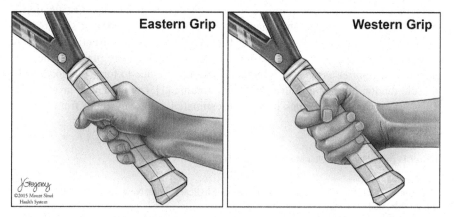

Fig. 9.1 Eastern grip versus Western grip. The pronated position of the hand in the Eastern grip is associated with radial-sided wrist pathologies, while the supinated position of the hand in the Western grip is associated with ulnar-sided wrist pain

The racket itself has also been studied. Hennig et al. showed that an increased racket head size and a higher resonance frequency were each associated with a decrease in arm vibration [8]. Athletes with oversized rackets had a lower incidence of injuries than those with conventional rackets. The mechanism may be that oversized rackets absorb the vibration from impacts better than conventional rackets and reduce the impact forces to the upper extremity [12]. However, the increase in weight of the racket can lead to higher torque forces, a tighter grip, and a higher incidence of injury.

Studies stress the importance of maintaining flexibility and strength in order to prevent injuries. The act of playing tennis may not actually strengthen the muscles required to prevent injury. As overload of muscle groups occur, the inflammation and tightening of these structures can lead to failure. A conditioning program is needed to prepare the young athlete's body for play. However, Kibler et al. noted in their study that despite a majority of young tennis players participating in flexibility programs, the incidence of inflexibility remained high. The ideal conditioning program may have yet to be elucidated, but knowledge of the patterns of injury will help in the design of such exercises [5].

Numerous studies point to risk factors that are specific to the young athlete. Muscle imbalances, low fitness level, and errors in training are commonly cited in the literature. Some studies have designed and implemented integrative neuromuscular training programs that have reduced the likelihood of sport-related injuries of both acute and overuse types by 15–50 % [13].

What Are the Injuries?

There is a broad spectrum of injuries that can occur with any young athlete ranging from bruises to fractures. The injuries that are more prevalent or clinically significant to the young tennis player will be discussed. However, the range of topics is by no means comprehensive and should preclude the reader from considering other possible diagnoses in the player.

Lateral Epicondylitis

Sometime in their career, approximately half of all competitive tennis players will suffer from tennis elbow [14, 15]. Tennis elbow, or lateral epicondylitis, most commonly refers to pain at the lateral epicondyle of the distal humerus. This is the site of the common extensor tendon origin and can be aggravated by repeated extension of the wrist. There are several theories as to the cause of lateral epicondylitis, with earlier literature attributing it to a chronic, degenerative tendinopathy featuring vascular proliferation and hyaline degeneration of the muscular origins of the extensor carpi radialis brevis and extensor digitorum communis [16]. Others hypothesize capsular involvement as well, suggesting a structural or anatomic predisposition. The radiocapitellar capsular complex is an outcropping of capsule surrounding the radial head, separate from the annular ligament, and which can become inflamed and hypertrophied. Both impingement of the radiocapitellar capsular complex and thickening of the plicae within the joint have been implicated as causes of lateral elbow pain [17, 18] (Fig. 9.2).

In average tennis players, the lateral epicondyle is problematic ten times more common than the medial epicondyle [19]. It has be postulated that a heavy racket, heavy balls, tight stringing, and grip size can lead to more stress at the lateral epicondyle [15]. Although not proven in clinical investigations, some authors believe that the incidence of lateral epicondylitis is lower in those with two-handed backhands as the nondominant arm is able to absorb some of the forces associated with the stroke. Also, using the second arm lessens the likelihood of faulty stroke mechanics [20, 21]. One investigation examined the muscle activity of the extensor

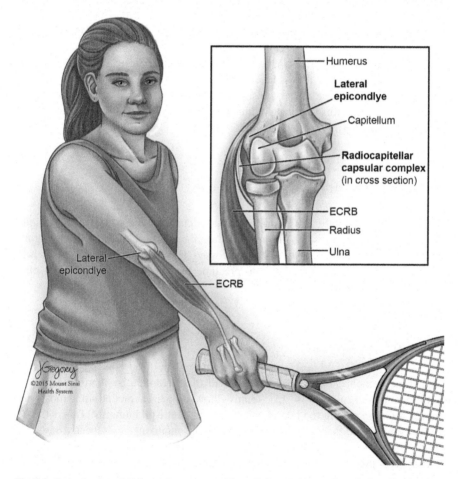

Fig. 9.2 Lateral epicondylitis can be aggravated by wrist extension, such as during a backswing. As shown in the inset picture, the site of pain is where the extensor carpi radialis brevis (*ECRB*), radiocapitellar capsular complex, and lateral epicondyle share a location

carpi radialis brevis between single and two-handed backhands, but did not show any significant differences in activity between the two strokes [22]. The use of vibration dampeners and changes in grip size have also been studied, but did not show an effect on the development of lateral epicondylitis [23–25]. In another study by Hennig et al., experienced tennis players were found to have reduced forearm vibration and decreased wrist extensor muscle activity during the backhand stroke when compared to novice players. The development of lateral epicondylitis is possibly more related to improper technique [8, 10].

Symptoms of lateral epicondylitis occur when the player grips tightly and extends the wrist causing pain at the elbow. There may be tenderness over the lateral epicondyle as well. Examination of the backstroke may reveal improper technique with too much motion at the wrist instead of the shoulder [19]. The player may also have limitations in wrist flexion compared to the contralateral extremity.

Treatment for lateral epicondylitis has focused on decreasing the inciting event with rest, corticosteroid injections to the site, and in refractory cases, arthroscopic debridement of the tendon in the operating room. Lateral epicondylitis usually resolves in the pediatric patient and persist symptoms may indicate the presence of a plica. Faulty stroke mechanics have been attributed as causes of lateral epicondylitis. The use of a doublehanded backhand stroke has a much lower incidence of lateral epicondylitis. The helping hand absorbs more energy and changes the mechanics of the swing [20, 21]. The player's nondominant hand prevents the leading wrist from hooking, helps to absorb impact and vibration, and provides the driving force for follow-through [21]. Therefore, it is often recommended that those players that cannot correct a faulty single-handed backhand be taught to use a doublehanded technique to prevent or aid treatment of an injury [22].

Medial Epicondylitis

Medial epicondylitis, often called golfer's elbow, is much less common than lateral epicondylitis, but can affect all athletes as the actions of flexion and pronation are common and inciting events if done repeatedly. In expert players, medial epicondylitis can be seen up to three times more commonly than lateral epicondylitis [19]. The medial epicondyle is the origination point of the flexor and pronator muscles of the forearm, with the pronator teres being a major contributor to topspin, particularly when using a Western or semi-Western grip which effectively forces supination in order to present the racket in the plane of the strings. This muscle force, combined with the valgus moment arm of the swing, can put a lot of stress on the medial aspect of the elbow. Repetitive strain on the muscle origin, bad stroke mechanics, or poor conditioning can all add to the trauma and cause microtearing.

Common symptoms are of medial elbow pain, exacerbated by playing time. However, the diagnostic picture can be clouded, as other causes of medial elbow pain can occur concomitantly with medial epicondylitis. Pathology such as ulnar collateral ligament injury, ulnar neuropraxia or cubital tunnel syndrome, and intra-articular injury can even occur in association. With the young tennis player, suspicion for a medial epicondyle apophysitis and avulsion should be high as will be discussed later. Other common symptoms include tenderness over the medial elbow and pain with resisted pronation [26].

Rest from play, ice, and nonsteroidal anti-inflammatory medications is believed to be useful for over 90 % of patients with medial epicondylitis. Nonsurgical treatment is usually successful, but surgical treatment can be of aid when a prolonged course of rehabilitation has failed to relieve symptoms [27].

Medial Epicondyle Apophysitis and Avulsion

Repetitive pulling forces over the medial elbow can lead to a distraction injury of the medial epicondyle apophysis. More commonly known to occur in little league pitchers, the valgus stress to the arm can put enormous stress on the ulnar collateral ligament which originates on the medial epicondyle apophysis [28]. Premature use of a heavier racquet may cause injury. Repetitive injury can lead to a progression of injury and pain. In the young athlete, ligaments are stronger than bone or growth plates. Therefore, as insult to the elbow continues, injury of the ulnar collateral ligament is rare compared to the bony injury of a medial epicondyle avulsion or injury at the tendon/bone junction, analogous to Osgood-Schlatter's disease of the knee.

Pain from medial epicondyle apophysitis and avulsion is very similar to medial epicondylitis and other medial elbow pathologies. There is pain over the medial elbow exacerbated by playing time and tenderness near the same area. When evaluating medial elbow pain, there should always be a suspicion for elbow instability. The stability of the elbow is provided by bony, ligamentous, and capsular structures. Therefore, when one component is injured, there should be an evaluation of other structures as well [29].

Treatment of medial epicondyle apophysitis is focused on rest, activity modification to avoid valgus stresses to the elbow, and gradual return to play as symptoms allow. If an avulsion has occurred, some advocate immediate surgical intervention for repair (Fig. 9.3).

Osteochondritis Dissecans

In skeletally immature athletes, valgus overload from excessive and overly forceful throwing or swinging can lead to capitellar osteochondritis dissecans (OCD) or Panner's disease, an avascular necrosis of the capitellum. Panner's disease is seen in children less than 10 years of age, presents as lateral elbow pain with restricted range of motion, and has a good prognosis if the offending activity is stopped. Capitellar OCD presents similarly to Panner's disease, but occurs in adolescents. It is associated with loose body formation, and except in young patients with no

Fig. 9.3 The medial epicondyle (*blue star*) has been avulsed from the humerus with widening of the growth plate. This may occur as the result of sudden trauma or may represent gradual failure of the apophysis due to chronic overloading

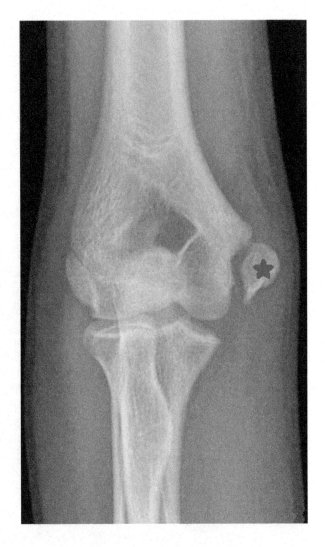

radiographic changes, operative treatment leads to better outcomes. Any athlete with pathologic changes in the lateral elbow from excess compressive forces should be examined for medial collateral ligament integrity.

Osteochondritis dissecans carries a poorer prognosis in patients with closed growth plates, but in a young patient, the prognosis is much more favorable. Off-loading the lesion by avoiding impact, rest, and refrain from play can possibly lead to healing of a stable, nondisplaced fragment. In young athletes who have undergone arthroscopic treatment of capitellar OCD or Panner's disease, short-term results are optimistic, with most patients returning to premorbid activity levels, including high-level throwing sports and gymnastics. Subjectively, patients report improved pain and increased range of motion [30, 31] (Fig. 9.4).

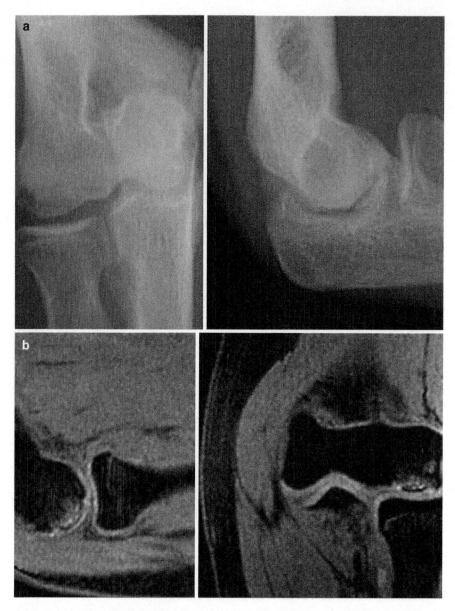

Fig. 9.4 An osteochondritis dissecans lesion. (**a**) The anteroposterior and lateral radiographs demonstrate capitellar lucency. (**b**) The sagittal and coronal T2 MR images demonstrate capitellar edema

Capitellar OCD lesions are amenable to arthroscopic treatment. Current surgical options include debridement, loose body excision, microfracture, chondral fixation, autologous bone graft, autologous osteochondral transplant, and autologous chondrocyte transplant. Most of these procedures involve an open approach, but arthroscopy is now playing a larger role with a less invasive approach. Arthroscopy allows better visualization of not only the radiocapitellar joint but also the other joints of the elbow, allowing for detection of accessory lesions (such as on the radial head, posterior capitellum, and trochlear notch of the capitellum) that may not be visible on conventional imaging or during an open approach [32]. Lesions amenable to arthroscopic debridement have been found in the anterior capitellum, posterolateral capitellum, and the posterior articular surface of the olecranon [33]. Loose bodies, reported in all compartments of the elbow, can be removed by arthroscopy [30]. Microfracturing through lateral portals has also been shown to be a viable treatment option, and if full range of motion is not obtained after debridement of lesions and loose bodies, arthroscopic capsulotomy may be performed.

An arthroscopic technique for the treatment of nondisplaced osteochondral fragments has been described [34]. A typical patient presents with lateral elbow pain and is diagnosed by physical examination, radiography, and MRI. The patient's symptoms did not improve with activity modification and nonoperative treatment. After visualization of the elbow and the lesion is done arthroscopically, the chondral defect is stabilized with a Freer elevator, while a guide wire for a cannulated drill is introduced from the posterior humerus into the center of the lesion. A tunnel, for introduction of bone graft and suture placement, is created over the guide wire with the cannulated drill (Fig. 9.5).

The patient is splinted in 90° of flexion for approximately 5 days and then started on range of motion exercises. Follow-up at 3 months showed painless, full range of motion, and radiographic healing. The author's technique provides a treatment solution of osteochondral defects using a less invasive approach and resulting in a quick recovery.

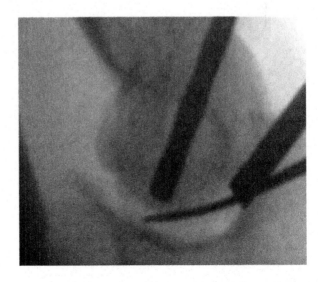

Fig. 9.5 The lateral radiograph shows a proximal anteromedial cannulated drill in the capitellum. A Freer elevator, the reduction, and the arthroscope enter the joint from the back

DeQuervain's Tenosynovitis

The most common tendinitis in racket sports is deQuervain's tenosynovitis [35]. In deQuervain's tenosynovitis, two main tendons of the thumb, the abductor pollicis longus and extensor pollicis brevis, have difficulty passing through a tunnel on the radial side of the wrist. Whether it is a thickening of the synovium surrounding the tendons or hypertrophy of the tunnel-like tendon sheath, the result is increased friction and pain with certain movements of the thumb and wrist.

Signs of deQuervain's tenosynovitis include pain along the radial side of the wrist, which can be exacerbated with forceful grasping of objects and twisting of the wrist. Swelling may be seen and the pain may travel up the forearm. The differential diagnosis can also include intersection syndrome or radial sensory neuritis (Fig. 9.6). Intersection syndrome is another form of overuse tenosynovitis, but occurs along the crossing of the abductor pollicis longus and extensor pollicis brevis tendons with the extensor carpi radialis longus and extensor carpi radialis brevis tendons. By also involving the abductor pollicis longus, the symptoms may overlap with deQuervain's tenosynovitis. With radial sensory neuritis, or Wartenberg's syndrome, the superficial branch of the radial nerve can become compressed between the muscles of the brachioradialis and the extensor carpi

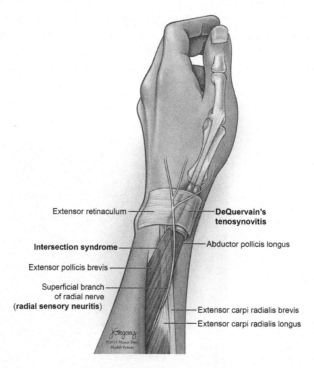

Fig. 9.6 Common pathologies for radial-sided wrist pain include deQuervain's tenosynovitis, intersection syndrome, and radial sensory neuritis

radialis longus. Symptoms can become worse with wrist pronation, such as with a tennis stroke, and include pain and paresthesias over the dorsoradial aspect of the hand.

Treatment of tenosynovitis is centered on rest and avoiding the activities that cause pain and swelling. Usually, rest from play for a few weeks will alleviate symptoms, with gradual return to play. Occasionally, recalcitrant symptoms may require splinting, corticosteroid injection, or surgery to release the tendon sheath.

Extensor Carpi Ulnaris Tendonitis

The extensor carpi ulnaris (ECU) is a tendon that travels alongside the ulnar head, inserting on the base of the fifth metacarpal, and is responsible for aiding extension and ulnar deviation of the wrist. ECU tendonitis is the second most common tendonitis in the athlete after deQuervain's tendonitis, possibly owing to forceful, sudden pronation to increase topspin [36]. It can be quite common in the nondominant wrist of the tennis player with a two-handed backhand. Biomechanical studies have shown that the nondominant wrist can be in excessive ulnar deviation during the two-handed backstroke [37, 38].

Signs of ECU tendonitis include weakness in grip strength, pain along the ulnar side of the wrist, and pain with wrist extension and ulnar deviation. Treatment involves rest, splinting, and anti-inflammatory medications. A corticosteroid injection can aid in reducing inflammation and symptoms, and stroke technique modifications are usually needed to prevent recurrence.

Extensor Carpi Ulnaris Subluxation

The ECU travels within an osteofibrous sheath as it passes the ulnar head. Subluxation of the ECU tendon can occur if this sheath has ruptured or attenuated. This can typically occur with a sudden forceful volar flexion and ulnar deviation of the wrist, such as when hitting a low forehand.

ECU subluxation can be diagnosed by having the athlete actively ulnarly deviates the wrist and slowly moves from full pronation to full supination. During this motion, the ECU tendon can be seen subluxing over the ulnar styloid [39]. If further aid in diagnosis is needed, a local anesthetic can be injected into the ECU tendon sheath, and relief of symptoms would be expected.

Treatment of ECU subluxation depends on the timing of the injury. In an acute injury, the arm can be casted for 6 weeks with the wrist pronated and extended [39, 40]. Open surgical repair can also be done with more predictable success and an earlier rehabilitation [41]. In chronic cases, reconstruction of the tendon sheath can give good results with eventual return to play [42].

Intersection Syndrome

Intersection syndrome is another inflammatory condition of the tendons across the wrist. The tendons involved are the abductor pollicis longus and extensor pollicis brevis crossing with the extensor carpi radialis longus and the extensor carpi radialis brevis. The intersection of these two groups of tendons is 46 cm proximal to the radiocarpal joint and is the location of the inflammation (Fig. 9.6).

The athlete typically presents with tenderness and swelling at the intersection point, and sometimes crepitus can be evidenced when the wrist is flexed and extended. Treatment is usually successful after a period of rest, splinting, and anti-inflammatory medications. If symptoms do not resolve, an injection of corticosteroids can be of aid or surgical decompression and debridement of the area [43]. Return to play is gradual once symptoms are relieved.

Triangular Fibrocartilage Complex Injuries

The triangular fibrocartilage complex (TFCC) is responsible for load transmission across the ulnocarpal joint as well as stability of the distal radioulnar joint. It is composed of a central articular disk portion that covers the ulnar head and radioulnar and ulnocarpal ligaments. Those with a positive ulnar variance have been shown to have increased injuries to the TFCC [44].

Patients with a TFCC injury often present with tenderness localized to the sulcus between the pisiform and the ulnar styloid. Pain may also be elicited with a supination lift test, piano key sign, or ulnar grind test. The complaints can range from a localized ulnar-sided wrist pain to a pain or discomfort throughout the entire wrist or distal forearm. Additionally, symptoms may overlap with other injuries such as extensor carpi ulnaris subluxation or injury, ulnar styloid fracture, and hamate fracture to name a few. An MRI can be useful in diagnosing and differentiation between these injuries. A CT or MRI scan can be used to assess distal radioulnar joint instability, which would warrant more urgent treatment.

Treatment of a TFCC tear is dependent on the severity of the injury. In a wrist with a stable distal radioulnar joint, initial treatment can consist of rest, splinting, and corticosteroid injections. If symptoms persist for 2–3 weeks, arthroscopic treatment ranging from debridement to repair of the TFCC may be indicated.

Hook of the Hamate Fracture

A fracture of the hook of the hamate can occur from a fall on an outstretched hand, repeated trauma due to impact from the butt of the tennis racket, or shearing forces from adjacent flexor tendons during forceful torquing of the wrist [45].

Symptoms include hypothenar pain, decreased grip strength, and tenderness to deep pressure over the hamate (Fig. 9.7). The most common symptom is pain with active grasp [46]. Since the ulnar nerve lies just medial to the hook of the hamate, the player may have symptoms of ulnar nerve impingement such as numbness and tingling on the medial one and a half fingers or weakness in pinching. Rarely, median nerve symptoms may also arise as the nerve lies lateral to the hook. Also lateral to the hook of the hamate is the tendon of the flexor digitorum profundus to the little finger, and tendinitis or rupture can occur in chronic cases. Pain with ring and little finger flexion that is worse with ulnar deviation and improved with radial deviation of the wrist can be indicative of an occult hook of the hamate injury with irritation of the flexor tendons [47]. An X-ray taken of the wrist in a carpal tunnel view will usually show the fracture. A computed tomography scan has been proven to be the most sensitive in detecting a hamate fracture [48].

An acute hook of the hamate fracture can usually be treated with immobilization in a short-arm cast. If the fracture fails to heal, excision or open reduction internal fixation of the fracture fragment can be done with satisfactory results with no clear advantage of one technique over the other [47, 49, 50]. A watershed area, where the vascular supply of the hamate can be vulnerable, has been proposed as contributing to the risk of nonunions of hook of the hamate fractures [51]. Return to sports is generally quick following excision of the hook, with scar sensitivity being the limiting factor [45].

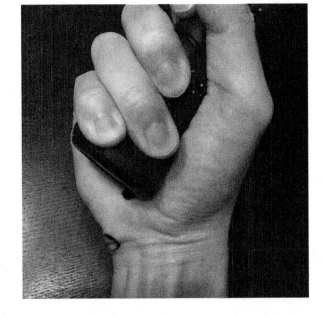

Fig. 9.7 The hook of the hamate is located at the dark circle. Note the proximity of the hook of the hamate to the end of the racket handle. To find the hook of the hamate, the distal thumb crease can be placed over the pisiform (*open circle*), and the tip of the thumb will fall onto the hook of the hamate

Arm Pump Syndrome

Chronic exertional compartment syndrome (CECS), or arm pump syndrome, is a condition in athletes that can occur after repetitive exertion. Common in moto-cross racers and long-distance runners, CECS can occur in any extremity, not just the more common lower leg. CECS is unlike acute compartment syndrome in that trauma is usually the cause of acute compartment syndrome. In CECS, elevated compartment pressures of the forearm remain elevated even after 30 min of cessation of exercise. Normally, pressures can normalize within 5 min of stopping. In CECS, however, the pressure remains high and impedes blood flow. As a result of decreased blood flow, the patient can experience muscle cramping and pain [52].

The onset of symptoms usually occurs at a specific time interval or intensity level of play. Feelings of pain are predominant, with possible weakness and paresthesias in the involved extremity. The symptoms usually subside after a period of inactivity and rest. The gold standard for diagnosis of CECS is compartment pressure measurements done during exercise and the period immediately following exercise.

Treatment for CECS is through surgical means. A conservative approach can be tried, but the results are usually recurrence with resumption of exercise. The surgical treatment is fascial release of the involved compartments and multiple techniques have been described [53]. The procedure can be performed in a minimally invasive, endoscopic manner, enabling athletes to return to their sport.

References

1. Kibler WB, McQueen C, Uhl T. Fitness evaluations and fitness findings in competitive junior tennis players. Clin Sports Med. 1988;7(2):403–16.
2. Beachy G, et al. High school sports injuries. A longitudinal study at Punahou School: 1988 to 1996. Am J Sports Med. 1997;25(5):675–81.
3. Hutchinson MR, et al. Injury surveillance at the USTA boys' tennis championships: a 6-yr study. Med Sci Sports Exerc. 1995;27(6):826–30.
4. Silva RT, et al. Medical assistance at the Brazilian juniors tennis circuit – a one-year prospective study. J Sci Med Sport. 2003;6(1):14–8.
5. Kibler WB, Safran MR. Musculoskeletal injuries in the young tennis player. Clin Sports Med. 2000;19(4):781–92.
6. Kitai E, et al. An epidemiological study of lateral epicondylitis (tennis elbow) in amateur male players. Ann Chir Main. 1986;5(2):113–21.
7. Jayanthi N, Sallay PI, Hunker P, et al. Skill-level related injuries in recreational competition tennis players. Med Sci Tennis. 2005;10:12–5.
8. Hennig EM, Rosenbaum D, Milani TL. Transfer of tennis racket vibrations onto the human forearm. Med Sci Sports Exerc. 1992;24(10):1134–40.
9. Wei SH, et al. Comparison of shock transmission and forearm electromyography between experienced and recreational tennis players during backhand strokes. Clin J Sport Med. 2006;16(2):129–35.
10. Abrams GD, Renstrom PA, Safran MR. Epidemiology of musculoskeletal injury in the tennis player. Br J Sports Med. 2012;46(7):492–8.

11. Tagliafico AS, et al. Wrist injuries in nonprofessional tennis players: relationships with different grips. Am J Sports Med. 2009;37(4):760–7.
12. Elliott BC, Blanksby BA, Ellis R. Vibration and rebound velocity characteristics of conventional and oversized tennis rackets. Res Q Exerc Sport. 1980;51(4):608–15.
13. Myer GD, et al. When to initiate integrative neuromuscular training to reduce sports-related injuries and enhance health in youth? Curr Sports Med Rep. 2011;10(3):155–66.
14. Maylack FH. Epidemiology of tennis, squash, and racquetball injuries. Clin Sports Med. 1988;7(2):233–43.
15. Pluim BM, et al. Tennis injuries: occurrence, aetiology, and prevention. Br J Sports Med. 2006;40(5):415–23.
16. Smith AM, Castle JA, Ruch DS. Arthroscopic resection of the common extensor origin: anatomic considerations. J Shoulder Elbow Surg. 2003;12(4):375–9.
17. Antuna SA, O'Driscoll SW. Snapping plicae associated with radiocapitellar chondromalacia. Arthroscopy. 2001;17(5):491–5.
18. Kim DH, et al. Arthroscopic treatment of posterolateral elbow impingement from lateral synovial plicae in throwing athletes and golfers. Am J Sports Med. 2006;34(3):438–44.
19. Kulund DN, et al. Tennis injuries: prevention and treatment. A review. Am J Sports Med. 1979;7(4):249–53.
20. Groppel JL, Nirschl RP. A mechanical and electromyographical analysis of the effects of various joint counterforce braces on the tennis player. Am J Sports Med. 1986;14(3):195–200.
21. Leach RE, Miller JK. Lateral and medial epicondylitis of the elbow. Clin Sports Med. 1987;6(2):259–72.
22. Giangarra CE, et al. Electromyographic and cinematographic analysis of elbow function in tennis players using single- and double-handed backhand strokes. Am J Sports Med. 1993;21(3):394–9.
23. De Smedt T, et al. Lateral epicondylitis in tennis: update on aetiology, biomechanics and treatment. Br J Sports Med. 2007;41(11):816–9.
24. Li FX, Fewtrell D, Jenkins M. String vibration dampers do not reduce racket frame vibration transfer to the forearm. J Sports Sci. 2004;22(11–12):1041–52.
25. Stroede CL, Noble L, Walker HS. The effect of tennis racket string vibration dampers on racket handle vibrations and discomfort following impacts. J Sports Sci. 1999;17(5):379–85.
26. Gabel GT, Morrey BF. Operative treatment of medial epicondylitis. Influence of concomitant ulnar neuropathy at the elbow. J Bone Joint Surg Am. 1995;77(7):1065–9.
27. Gregg JR, Torg E. Upper extremity injuries in adolescent tennis players. Clin Sports Med. 1988;7(2):371–85.
28. Gill 4th TJ, Micheli LJ. Common injuries and overuse syndromes of the elbow and wrist. Clin Sports Med. 1996;15(2):401–23.
29. Ciccotti MC, Schwartz MA, Ciccotti MG. Diagnosis and treatment of medial epicondylitis of the elbow. Clin Sports Med. 2004;23(4):693–705, xi.
30. Krijnen MR, Lim L, Willems WJ. Arthroscopic treatment of osteochondritis dissecans of the capitellum: report of 5 female athletes. Arthroscopy. 2003;19(2):210–4.
31. Takahara M, et al. Classification, treatment, and outcome of osteochondritis dissecans of the humeral capitellum. J Bone Joint Surg Am. 2007;89(6):1205–14.
32. Robla J, et al. Chondromalacia of the trochlear notch in athletes who throw. J Shoulder Elbow Surg. 1996;5(1):69–72.
33. Bojanic I, Ivkovic A, Boric I. Arthroscopy and microfracture technique in the treatment of osteochondritis dissecans of the humeral capitellum: report of three adolescent gymnasts. Knee Surg Sports Traumatol Arthrosc. 2006;14(5):491–6.
34. Hsu JW, et al. The emerging role of elbow arthroscopy in chronic use injuries and fracture care. Hand Clin. 2009;25(3):305–21.
35. Posner MA. Injuries to the hand and wrist in athletes. Orthop Clin North Am. 1977;8(3):593–618.
36. Wood MB, Dobyns JH. Sports-related extraarticular wrist syndromes. Clin Orthop Relat Res. 1986;202:93–102.

37. Rettig AC. Wrist problems in the tennis player. Med Sci Sports Exerc. 1994;26(10):1207–12.
38. Rettig AC. Athletic injuries of the wrist and hand: part II: overuse injuries of the wrist and traumatic injuries to the hand. Am J Sports Med. 2004;32(1):262–73.
39. Taleisnik J. The ligaments of the wrist. J Hand Surg Am. 1976;1(2):110–8.
40. Burkhart SS, Wood MB, Linscheid RL. Posttraumatic recurrent subluxation of the extensor carpi ulnaris tendon. J Hand Surg Am. 1982;7(1):1–3.
41. Rowland SA. Acute traumatic subluxation of the extensor carpi ulnaris tendon at the wrist. J Hand Surg Am. 1986;11(6):809–11.
42. MacLennan AJ, et al. Diagnosis and anatomic reconstruction of extensor carpi ulnaris subluxation. J Hand Surg Am. 2008;33(1):59–64.
43. Grundberg AB, Reagan DS. Pathologic anatomy of the forearm: intersection syndrome. J Hand Surg Am. 1985;10(2):299–302.
44. Palmer AK, Werner FW. Biomechanics of the distal radioulnar joint. Clin Orthop Relat Res. 1984;187:26–35.
45. Marchessault J, Conti M, Baratz ME. Carpal fractures in athletes excluding the scaphoid. Hand Clin. 2009;25(3):371–88.
46. Bishop AT, Beckenbaugh RD. Fracture of the hamate hook. J Hand Surg Am. 1988;13(1):135–9.
47. Walsh 4th JJT, Bishop AT. Diagnosis and management of hamate hook fractures. Hand Clin. 2000;16(3):397–403, viii.
48. Andresen R, et al. Imaging of hamate bone fractures in conventional X-rays and high-resolution computed tomography. An in vitro study. Invest Radiol. 1999;34(1):46–50.
49. Hirano K, Inoue G. Classification and treatment of hamate fractures. Hand Surg. 2005;10(2–3):151–7.
50. Scheufler O, et al. Hook of hamate fractures: critical evaluation of different therapeutic procedures. Plast Reconstr Surg. 2005;115(2):488–97.
51. Failla JM. Hook of hamate vascularity: vulnerability to osteonecrosis and nonunion. J Hand Surg Am. 1993;18(6):1075–9.
52. Reneman RS. The anterior and the lateral compartmental syndrome of the leg due to intensive use of muscles. Clin Orthop Relat Res. 1975;113:69–80.
53. Black KP, Taylor DE. Current concepts in the treatment of common compartment syndromes in athletes. Sports Med. 1993;15(6):408–18.

Chapter 10
Tennis Injuries of the Hip and Knee

Steven M. Andelman and Alexis C. Colvin

Introduction

Extensive efforts to both quantify and qualify injuries common to the young tennis athlete have come to represent a growing body of literature with contributions from multiple specialists including orthopedic surgeons, physiatrists, athletic trainers, and biomechanical scientists. Early research into the subject focused mainly on epidemiologic studies, attempting to enumerate the most common injuries encountered in competitive youth tennis. Later research concentrated on describing the etiology, diagnosis, and treatment of tennis-specific injuries. The majority of these efforts have focused on conditions of the upper extremity at the elbow and shoulder. It has not been until recently that interest has turned toward the unique biomechanical, anatomic, and pathologic stresses placed on the hip and knee during tennis.

This chapter will serve as a review of the literature of injuries to the hip and knee encountered in the young tennis athlete. Following the trend of the available literature, this review will begin with analysis of the numerous attempts to describe the epidemiology of injuries to the lower extremities within various populations of tennis athletes. The focus will then shift toward the specific injuries of the hip and knee seen in young tennis athletes and end with future directions for research.

S.M. Andelman, MD (✉) • A.C. Colvin, MD
Department of Orthopaedic Surgery,
Mount Sinai Medical Center,
New York, NY, USA
e-mail: steve.andelman@gmail.com

© Springer International Publishing Switzerland 2016
A.C. Colvin, J.N. Gladstone (eds.), *The Young Tennis Player: Injury Prevention and Treatment*, Contemporary Pediatric and Adolescent Sports Medicine,
DOI 10.1007/978-3-319-27559-8_10

183

Epidemiology of Tennis Injuries

Many early attempts at characterizing tennis injuries were aimed at determining their incidence in different age groups at varying levels of play. A comprehensive 2006 review of literature regarding injuries associated with tennis identified 31 total epidemiologic studies from 1966 to 2006 [1]. These ranged from small prospective studies of elite-level athletes to large, survey-based retrospective studies of recreational-level players. In addition to the variety of studies, each set of authors also provided differing definitions of what constitutes an "injury," thus leading to conflicting levels of reported incidence. Table 10.1 provides a sample of the available literature and demonstrates the variability of study structure as well as the associated inconsistency in the reported results.

Hutchinson et al. followed 1440 participants in the United States Tennis Association (USTA) Boy's Tennis Championships over 6 years and reported an injury rate of 21.5/1000 athletic exposures, with one athletic exposure equivalent to a tennis match [5]. Contrast this to Winge et al. who followed 89 elite-level young male and female athletes over one tennis season and reported 2.3 injuries/1000 h of tennis [3]. Assuming the relative comparability between "athletic exposures" and "hours of tennis," this nearly tenfold difference can most likely be attributed to the strict definition of an injury by Winge in comparison to that used by Hutchinson. Winge defined an injury as that which "handicapped" an athlete or required "special attention" from medical personnel, while Hutchinson defined an injury as anything requiring medical assistance.

Better clarity, especially from the perspective of the treating physician, can come from studies with a more strict definition of injury. Defining an injury as that which prevented tennis play for greater than seven days, Jayanthi et al. reported an incidence of 3.0 injuries/1000 h [9]. Similarly, Lanese et al. prospectively followed 12 male and 11 female college-level athletes monitoring for injuries that prevented participation in competitive play and reported an incidence of 1.6 and 1.0 injuries/1000 h, respectively [4]. Corroborating the results of these early epidemiologic studies, Hjelm et al. reported a rate of 1.7 and 0.6 injuries/1000 h of tennis for male and female athletes, respectively [9]. Using a more strict definition of "injury" as an incident that causes an athlete to be unable to compete, the true incidence of injury for both recreational and competitive tennis players likely lies between 0.6 and 3.0 injuries/1000 h as reported above.

To put the incidence of tennis-related injuries in young athletes into context, they can be compared to reported rates of injury for other common sports. Hootman et al. published 16 years of data on collegiate injuries sustained during practice and competitive events [12]. In this retrospective review, an injury was defined as that which caused an athlete to miss at least one day of competitive play. All data was expressed in terms of "athlete events" (AE), defined as the participation of one athlete in one practice or game. Reported rates of injury ranged from 35.9 injuries/1000 AE in men's football to 4.3 injuries/1000 AE in women's softball. While this data was expressed in terms of "athletic events," and not in "hours of sport"

Table 10.1 Selected epidemiologic publications on tennis injuries

Study	Format	Population	Number	Definition of injury	Incidence of injury
Reece [2]	Retrospective	Elite tennis athletes ages 16–20	45	An injury that required medical attention from a physician or athletic trainer	M: 2.5 injuries/player/year F: 2.9 injuries/player/year
Winge [3]	Prospective	Elite M + F Danish young tennis athletes	89	An injury that handicapped an athlete or required special treatment	Total: 2.3 injuries/1000 h of tennis M: 2.7 injuries/1000 h F: 1.1 injuries/1000 h
Lanese et al. [4]	Prospective	M + F college athletes	23	Any injury resulting in absence of play	M: 1.6 injuries/1000 h F: 1.0 injury/1000 h
Hutchinson [5]	Retrospective	USTA boys championship < 18 years old	1440	All injuries that required medical attention	9.9 new injuries/100 athletes 21.5 injuries/1000 athletic exposures
Hahn [6]	Retrospective	Danish competitive athletes 14–35	339	Any knee pain in preceding 12 months	42.5 % with knee pain 15 % with absence due to pain
Sallis [7]	Retrospective	Mixed sport M + F college athletes 18–22	3767 total athletes, injuries separated by sport, no sport-specific "N" given	An injury that required attention of athletic trainer	M: 0.465 injuries/player/year F: 0.425 injury/player/year
Silva [8]	Prospective	Brazilian junior tennis circuit M + F 12–18	258	Any consultation or treatment given to an athlete during a tournament	6.9 medical treatments/1000 games played
Jayanthi [9]	Retrospective questionnaire	M + F recreational tennis players	428	Any injury preventing play for > 7 days	3.0 injuries/1000 h
Hjelm [10]	Prospective	Swedish competitive tennis players 12–18	55	An injury that makes it impossible to participate in regular tennis on at least 1 occasion	M: 1.7 injuries/1000 h F: 0.6 injury/1000 h

Table partially modified from Pluim et al. [1] and Abrams et al. [11].

Table 10.2 Common sites of tennis-related injuries

Study	% Lower extremity	% Upper extremity	% Trunk	% Knee injuries	% Hip injuries
Reece [2]	59 %	20 %	21 %	–	–
Winge [3]	39 %	46 %	24 %	4.3 %	–
Hutchinson [5]	49 %	26 %	25 %	19.2 %	8.8 %
Sallis et al. [7]	M: 62.2 % F: 70.7 %	M: 23.1 % F: 21.9 %	M: 14.6 % F: 7.2 %	M: 6.11 % F: 11.0 %	M: 3.7 % F: 8.5 %
Jayanthi et al. [9]	41 %	43 %	11 %	12 %	5 % *
Hjelm [10]	50 %	25 %	25 %	14 %	5 % **

*denoted as thigh/groin strain
**denoted as groin strain

Table 10.3 Common types of tennis-related injuries

Study	Mechanism of injury
Winge [3]	Sprain: 17 % Strain: 14 % Fracture: 2 %
Hutchinson [5]	Sprain: 58 % Strain: 21 % Contusion: 7 %
Silva et al. [8]	Muscle contracture: 26 % Strain: 11 % Sprain: 6 %

such as the aforementioned epidemiologic data for tennis injuries, it is appropriate to assume that tennis has a relatively low injury rate when compared to other common sports.

A subset of the epidemiologic studies also reported on the location and type of injury sustained during tennis play. Table 10.2 represents a review of the location of injury with special attention to the hip and knee. Although differences exist, the majority of data suggests that lower extremity injuries predominate with approximately twice as many injuries occurring at the knee compared to the hip.

Of those studies that reported on etiology of injury, chronic injuries are shown to be more common than acute injuries [3, 9, 10]. Looking specifically at acute injuries, sprains, strains, and muscular contusions occur with relative frequency, while fractures and ligamentous tears were rarely reported (Table 10.3). Only Hjelm looked specifically at mechanism of injury, reporting that 30 % of all injuries occurred while hitting a ball, 24 % occurred during training exercises, 9 % were attributed to twisting injuries, and 5 % were attributed to acceleration/deceleration movements [10].

Overall, the epidemiologic studies of injuries in young tennis athletes reveal a relatively low incidence of injury with a predominance of chronic injuries over acute occurring most frequently in the lower extremities.

Development and Anatomy of the Hip and Knee

A basic understanding of the development and anatomy of the hip and knee is essential prior to discussion of common lower extremity injuries seen in young tennis athletes.

The knee is composed of two articulations – tibiofemoral and patellofemoral. The tibiofemoral articulation is a ginglymus or "hinge-type" articulation that allows for rotation as well as flexion and extension in the sagittal plane. The tibiofemoral articulation functions to transmit forces from the femur to the tibia. Stability to the tibiofemoral articulation is derived from the surrounding ligamentous and tendinous structures. The medial and lateral collateral ligaments resist valgus and varus stress, respectively, while the anterior cruciate ligament is the primary restraint to anterior translation of the tibia on the femur, and the posterior cruciate ligament is the primary restraint to posterior translation of the tibia on the femur. Multiple other dynamic stabilizers play a role in tibiofemoral function including the gastrocnemius, popliteus, and hamstring muscles. In the developing skeleton two primary physes are present – one at the distal femur and one at the proximal tibia. These two physes allow for the highest rate of longitudinal growth in the body with the distal femoral physis growing at a rate of 0.9 mm/year and the proximal tibial physis growing at a rate of 0.6 mm/year [13]. Closure of the distal femoral and proximal tibial physes occurs at the onset of skeletal maturity, considered to be between 13 and 14 years of age in females and 15–16 years of age in males [13] (Fig. 10.1).

The patellofemoral joint is a gliding articulation that functions to transmit forces from the quadriceps tendon to the patellar tendon to facilitate extension of the tibiofemoral joint. The patella sits within the trochlea of the distal femur. The quadriceps tendon inserts on the superior pole of the patella, while the patellar tendon originates at the inferior pole of the patella and inserts distally on the tibial tubercle. Further stability of patellar motion is derived from the insertions of the vastus medialis and lateralis as well as the medial patellofemoral ligament. The primary structure of importance in the developing skeleton is the tibial tubercle apophysis into which the patellar tendon inserts. This secondary growth center is cartilaginous up until age 11 after which an apophysis begins to form that is visible on radiographic examination. Apophyseal maturation occurs from age 11 to 14. From age 14 to 18, the apophysis fuses with the tibial epiphysis, and after age 18 the fused epiphysis and apophysis fuse to the rest of the tibia [14].

The hip is a ball-and-socket joint with the proximal femoral head articulating into the acetabulum. The hip allows for multidirectional movement including flexion, extension, adduction, abduction, and internal and external rotation. Hip stability and motion is determined both by the bony articulation between the femoral head and the acetabulum as well as the many dynamic stabilizing muscles that cross the hip joint including the gluteus medius and minimus (abduction); the adductor magnus, longus, and brevis (adduction); the gluteus maximus (extension); the iliopsoas (flexion); and the short external rotator muscles (external rotation). Further

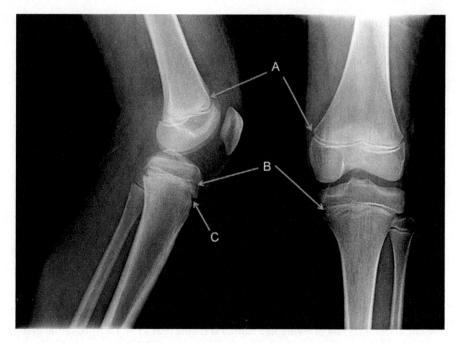

Fig. 10.1 Lateral and AP radiographs of the pediatric knee. (*A*) Distal femoral physis, (*B*) proximal tibial physis, (*C*) tibial tubercle apophysis, and attachment of the patellar tendon

stability comes from the hip labrum, analogous to the labrum of the shoulder, which provides a deepening of the acetabular socket.

The developing pediatric hip is composed of multiple ossification centers that arise at varying ages. While the femoral shaft and femoral capital epiphysis are present at birth, the femoral head appears at 4–6 months of age, the greater trochanter appears at 2–4 years of age, and the lesser trochanter appears later during puberty [15]. All ossification centers fuse after the onset of puberty between 14 and 18 years of age. The acetabulum is composed of the triradiate cartilage that represents the confluence of the ilium, ischium, and pubic innominate bones. Not a true secondary center of ossification, the triradiate cartilage fuses between 14 and 18 years of age [16, 17] (Fig. 10.2).

Knee Injuries

From a biomechanical perspective, tennis places a high level of stress on the knee joint and surrounding ligamentous and tendinous stabilizing structures. Tennis play requires short bursts of high-intensity running interspersed with the stopping, starting, pivoting, and twisting motions necessary to reach the location of the ball, maneuver to set up the impending stroke, and return the ball to the opponent. The

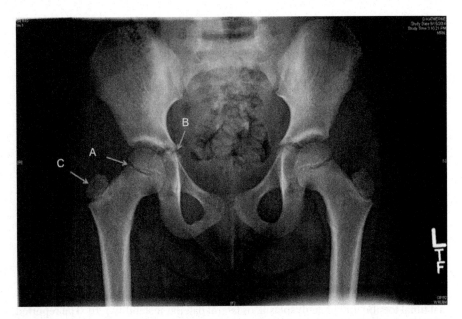

Fig. 10.2 AP radiograph of the pediatric hip. (*A*) Proximal femoral physis, (*B*) apophysis of the greater trochanter, (*C*) triradiate cartilage

average tennis point involves more than eight changes of direction, each placing a load of 1.5–2.7 times the involved body weight through the knee joint and surrounding structures [18]. Available data suggests that 4.3–19.2 % of all tennis-related injuries occur to the knee [3, 5, 8, 9]. While the majority of tennis injuries in young athletes tend to be chronic overuse injuries to the patellofemoral compartment and extensor mechanism, the twisting and pivoting motions necessary for tennis play produce a unique profile of injuries to the tendinous and ligamentous stabilizing structures of the knee.

Chronic Knee Pain

A significant amount of knee injuries encountered in young tennis athletes have been characterized as "overuse" injuries [2–4]. The repetitive knee flexion and extension during tennis play leads to microtrauma to the knee joint. Published rates of chronic knee injuries have varied from 30 to 72 % [5, 10, 19]. The majority of these injuries can be localized to the extensor mechanism and patellofemoral compartment with patellofemoral pain syndrome, quadriceps and patellar tendonitis, Osgood-Schlatter's disease (OSD), iliotibial band (ITB) syndrome, and bursitis being the most commonly encountered diagnoses [10, 23, 37]. There have been few attempts to determine the true incidence of the each individual diagnosis. Hjelm et al. reported on 14 chronic knee injuries out of 100 total injuries. Within this subset, the authors reported on one case of patellofemoral pain syndrome (7 %), three cases of patellar or quadriceps tendinopathy (21 %), two cases of ITB syndrome (14 %), and two cases of OSD (14 %) [10].

Differentiating between causes of chronic knee pain and arriving at a single diagnosis can be difficult due to the subtle differences of presentation between the varying pathologies. The following represents an overview of the most common causes of chronic knee pain in young tennis athletes including etiology, diagnosis, and initial treatment modalities.

Patellofemoral Pain Syndrome

Patellofemoral pain syndrome (idiopathic chondromalacia patellae) is characterized by aching anterior knee pain exacerbated by knee flexion. Pain is caused by maltracking of the patella within the trochlear groove leading to abnormal forces within the patellofemoral compartment. It can arise due to a multitude of intrinsic anatomic factors including a high "q angle" caused by increased femoral anteversion or external tibial torsion, trochlear dysplasia, or lateral patellar instability [20]. The reported incidence of patellofemoral pain syndrome in young tennis athletes is between 7 and 16 % [10, 21]. It is important to note that patellofemoral pain syndrome is due to inherent anatomic variations to the patellofemoral compartment that are exacerbated by the repetitive knee flexion required by tennis play (Fig. 10.3).

Patellofemoral pain syndrome is a difficult diagnosis to make and is many times considered a diagnosis of exclusion. Presence of obvious anatomic causes as

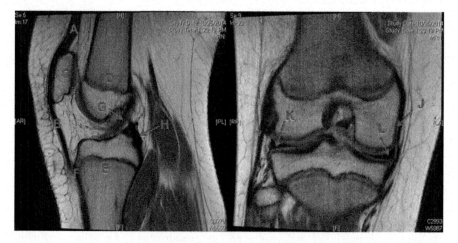

Fig. 10.3 Sagittal and coronal views of the pediatric knee. (*A*) Quadriceps tendon, (*B*) patellar tendon, (*C*) patella, (*D*) distal femoral physis, (*E*) proximal tibial physis, (*F*) insertion of patellar tendon into tibial tubercle apophysis, (*G*) anterior cruciate ligament, (*H*) posterior cruciate ligament, (*I*) lateral collateral ligament, (*J*) medial collateral ligament, (*K*) lateral meniscus, (*L*) medial meniscus

described above as seen on either x-ray or advanced imaging facilitates such a task. In the absence of such findings, many patients will complain of generalized anterior knee pain without point tenderness. Patients may complain of pain with other actions requiring deep knee flexion such as navigation of stairs. If a diagnosis of patellofemoral pain syndrome is suspected, initial treatment always involves rest, nonsteroidal anti-inflammatory medications, and long-term physical therapy directed toward core and quadriceps strengthening [22].

Quadriceps and Patellar Tendonitis

Quadriceps and patellar tendonitis occur at the insertion of the quadriceps tendon at the superior pole of the patella and the origin of the patellar tendon at the inferior pole of the patella, respectively. Both diagnoses are seen often in sports requiring knee flexion and extension due to repetitive eccentric contractions of the extensor mechanism leading to microtears at the bone-tendon interface [21, 23]. Quadriceps and patellar tendonitis are thus understandably seen in young tennis athletes given the repetitive deep knee flexion and extension necessary to complete a tennis stroke.

While both quadriceps and patellar tendonitis cause diffuse anterior knee pain, they can be differentiated by location of point tenderness and exacerbating maneuvers. Whereas quadriceps tendonitis will lead to pain with palpation of the superior pole of the patella and be exacerbated with knee extension, patellar tendonitis will lead to pain with palpation of the inferior pole of the patella and be exacerbated with knee flexion. Clinical examination is usually sufficient to diagnose quadriceps and patellar tendonitis. However, knee ultrasound and magnetic resonance imaging (MRI) can help confirm diagnosis or aide in diagnosing more subtle presentations.

Treatment is based on conservative measures including rest, nonsteroidal anti-inflammatory medications, and physical therapy initiated upon resolution of pain directed first at range of motion exercises before progressing to loading of the quadriceps mechanism [24, 25].

Osgood-Schlatter's Disease (OSD)

Osgood-Schlatter's disease (tibial tubercle traction apophysitis) is another common cause of pain in adolescent athletes who participate in sports that involve jumping or flexion activities. It arises due to repetitive tension placed on the insertion of the patellar tendon at the apophysis of the tibial tubercle in skeletally immature patients prior to fusion between the apophysis and tibial epiphysis. Repetitive traction forces placed on the unfused apophysis lead to point tenderness and pain over the tibial tubercle. In this manner OSD can be seen as analogous to patellar tendonitis in skeletally immature tennis athletes [26].

Diagnosis of OSD is made purely on a clinical basis in skeletally immature patients with tibial tubercle tenderness associated with knee flexion. Imaging rarely plays a role in diagnosis, although x-ray imaging can demonstrate irregularity of the tibial tubercle [27].

Like patellar tendonitis, initial treatment is conservative and aimed at rest, nonsteroidal anti-inflammatory medications, and physical therapy directed at quadriceps stretching to decrease tension on the unfused apophysis. Recalcitrant cases can be treated with an extended period of long leg cast immobilization or, if skeletally mature, excision of any residual fragmented ossicles of the tibial tubercle [28] (Fig. 10.4).

Iliotibial Band Friction Syndrome

Iliotibial band (ITB) syndrome arises from excessive friction between the ITB and lateral femoral condyle. It has been associated with a variety of anatomic and physiologic abnormalities including weak hip abductors, a tight ITB, increased tibial

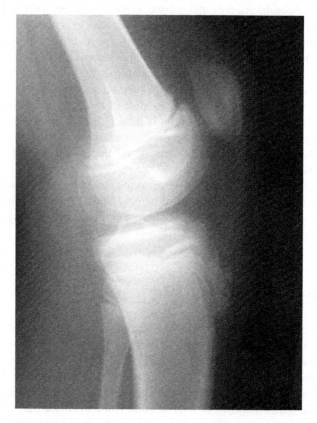

Fig. 10.4 Lateral radiograph of the knee demonstrating tibial tubercle apophyseal irregularities associated with OSD [29]

internal rotation, genu varum, and mismatch between hamstring and quadriceps strength – all of which can cause maltracking of the ITB and irritation at the area overlying the lateral femoral condyle. ITB friction syndrome is seen commonly in sports that require repetitive knee flexion and extension such as cycling and running as well as in those athletes who undergo a sudden, rapid increase in training intensity [30]. ITB friction syndrome has been identified in young tennis athletes, especially at the onset of training during preseason conditioning [21].

Diagnosis of ITB friction syndrome can be made clinically with point tenderness over the lateral femoral condyle in the region of the ITB with reproduction of pain with deep knee flexion. The Ober test can help to identify ITB pathology. In this maneuver the patient is placed lateral lying on the unaffected side. The affected knee is brought from flexion and abduction to extension and adduction. Decreased ability to adduct is suggestive of ITB tightness, while pain during the maneuver is suggestive of ITB inflammation. Radiographs and MRI do not so much aide in diagnosis as help to identify possible underlying anatomic abnormalities and rule out lateral knee compartment intraarticular pathology [30].

After a diagnosis of ITB friction syndrome, conservative treatment is initiated with a focus on stretching the ITB and strengthening hip abductors. In the rare instance of recalcitrant ITB friction syndrome, corticosteroid injections have proven effective. Surgical ITB lengthening represents an option of last resort after all conservative measures have failed [30].

Bursitis

There are multiple bursas about the knee that can become irritated and inflamed from the flexion, twisting, and pivoting motions that occur throughout a tennis match. The most commonly encountered diagnoses are prepatellar bursitis, pes anserinus bursitis, and semimembranosus bursitis [21]. There is no published literature concerning the incidence of these injuries in young tennis athletes. Diagnosis of bursitis is clinical and based on tenderness to the bursa in question and pain with associated provocative movements. Treatment is aimed at conservative management with rest and nonsteroidal anti-inflammatory medications with corticosteroid injections relegated for those patients unresponsive to more conservative measures.

Acute Knee Injuries

Acute ligamentous injuries of the knee are less common than chronic overuse injuries. Reported incidence of acute knee injuries varies widely depending on the definition of injury, with published rates ranging from 28 to 70 % [10, 19]. The most common types of acute knee injuries are ligamentous "sprains," representing

6–58 % of all knee injuries, although there is no specification as to which knee structure is injured in these studies [3, 5, 8, 10]. Historically, the medial collateral ligament (MCL) was the most frequently injured knee structure in tennis [18, 21]; however there is little published data on tennis injuries to the MCL. Based on the available data, the medial meniscus is the most frequently injured structure followed by the anterior cruciate ligament (ACL) and lateral meniscus [31, 32].

Intraarticular Knee Injuries

A review of 129 tennis-related knee injuries as a subset of over 3000 sport-related intraarticular injuries over a 10-year period diagnosed via MRI or arthroscopy revealed 66 injuries to the medial meniscus, 33 ACL injuries, and 19 lateral meniscal injuries, while only two injuries to the MCL were noted [31]. The 51.2 % incidence of medial meniscal injuries was nearly five times the 10.8 % average incidence of medial meniscal injury across all sports reviewed. In contrast to the high rate of meniscal injuries, tennis was associated with a relatively low rate of injuries to the ACL. ACL injuries were the most common pathology encountered across all sports, diagnosed in 45 % of all subjects. This is nearly double the 26 % incidence of ACL injuries encountered in tennis athletes. This data confirms an earlier review of 128 arthroscopies performed for injuries sustained during racquet sports, including tennis, which reported a 36 % incidence of meniscal injury and a 10.8 % incidence of ACL injury [32].

As tennis is a noncontact sport dependent on repetitive pivoting and twisting motions throughout a given match, a predominance of injuries to the menisci and a relatively low rate of injuries to the ACL are consistent with regular tennis play. However, it is important to note that both aforementioned studies involve athletes of all ages and do not focus solely on young tennis players. It is generally felt that young tennis athletes have a relatively low rate of intraarticular ligamentous injuries [18, 19] (Fig. 10.5).

Diagnosis of intraarticular knee injuries should be guided by clinical exam with MRI used only for confirmatory purposes. Differentiation between meniscal and ACL injuries can be challenging. Injuries to the ACL are usually associated with an immediate large knee effusion, while the relatively avascular nature of the meniscus causes more subtle effusions. Patients with an ACL injury will complain of knee instability and will have increased anterior translation of the proximal tibia on the distal femur during anterior drawer and Lachman testing. In contrast, patients with meniscal injuries will likely complain more often of locking or mechanical knee symptoms with associated tenderness to palpation over the affected tibial plateau joint line [33].

A full discussion of the treatment of intraarticular knee injuries in tennis is beyond the scope of this chapter. Broadly, decisions regarding treatment should take into account the age, competitive level, associated injuries, injury type, patient preference, and surgeon expertise.

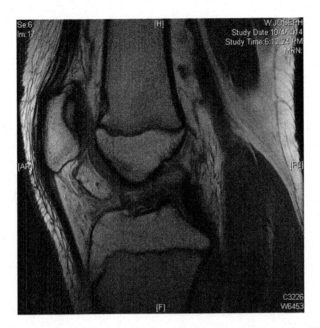

Fig. 10.5 Sagittal view of pediatric knee demonstrating a tear of anterior cruciate ligament

Tennis Leg

Tennis leg is an eponym for an acute muscular strain or tear at the myotendinous origin of the medial head of the gastrocnemius [34, 35]. This injury occurs with sudden transition from ankle plantar flexion to dorsiflexion with the knee in extension, as seen on the back leg during the tennis serve [36, 37]. Originally described in adult and recreational athletes, tennis leg is felt to be relatively uncommon in young tennis players [19].

Diagnosis is based on a compelling history of injury with tenderness over the course of the medial head of the gastrocnemius muscle, more commonly occurring in the proximal half of the muscle belly. MRI can be used as an adjunct to confirm suspected diagnosis demonstrating inflammation along the muscle belly. As with the chronic knee injuries described above, treatment is conservative with an initial period of rest and nonsteroidal anti-inflammatory medications followed by physical therapy for range of motion and strengthening exercises.

Hip Injuries

The hip and pelvis play an essential role in tennis in generating the rotational torque necessary to allow for transmission of power from the lower extremities to the upper extremities and eventually through the swinging racquet. Biomechanical studies

Fig. 10.6 Schematic
representation of the major
muscular stabilizers of the
hip joint. The adductors
are a common site of
injuries in young tennis
athletes [39]

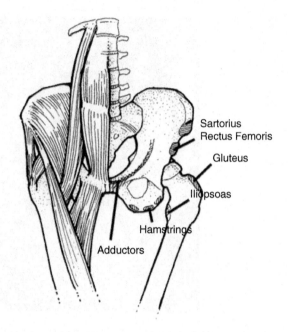

Sartorius
Rectus Femoris

Gluteus

Iliopsoas

Hamstrings

Adductors

have demonstrated that the trunk and pelvis rotate at 350°/s [18] with an associated pelvic angular displacement of 54–60° throughout the backhand and forehand strokes [38]. Generation of such movements is reliant on hip adduction at the front or leading leg and hip extension at the back leg, with subtle differences dependent on stroke type [38]. An understanding of the forces transmitted through the hip provides a starting point for studying the injury patterns to the hip in young tennis athletes (Fig. 10.6).

Adductor Muscle Strains

Available data suggests that the incidence of hip injuries, including injuries to the "groin," represents 3.7–8.8 % of all tennis-related injuries [5, 7, 10]. The majority of all documented injuries to the hip are adductor muscle strains. Empirically, this is felt to be due to the extreme leg abduction that can occur while reaching for a ball in the "split" position. The high incidence of adductor strains is further explained by the lead hip adduction observed during the tennis stroke as discussed above.

Diagnosis and treatment are similar as for strains of the medial head of the gastrocnemius. Diagnosis is clinical with pain over the medial hip at the insertion of the adductors. Treatment is conservative and based on limiting abduction, nonsteroidal anti-inflammatory medications, and gradual return to play.

Intraarticular Injuries

In the aforementioned epidemiologic studies, there have been no attempts to describe hip injuries in young tennis athletes beyond "sprains" and "strains" to the groin. Recently, there have been endeavors to characterize the effects of tennis play on both hip rotation and the dynamic stabilizing muscles of the hip joint given the repetitive asymmetric loading of the hip during tennis.

Using MRI in to characterize the major stabilizers of the hip joint, Sanchis-Moysi et al. found that young, elite tennis athletes had asymmetric hypertrophy of the nondominant (back leg) iliopsoas and symmetric hypertrophy of the gluteal muscles when compared to control subjects [40]. However, asymmetric differences in the dynamic stabilizers of the hip do not appear to affect hip rotation. Ellenbecker et al. described the normative hip internal and external rotation values for 147 young, elite male and female tennis athletes and found no statistically significant difference in internal or external rotation between the dominant and nondominant hips [41]. While there may not be differences in dominant and nondominant hip rotation in asymptomatic patients, Vad et al. found a statistically significant decrease in dominant hip internal rotation in tennis athletes with self-reported low back pain [42].

While differences in muscle development can exist between the dominant and nondominant hips, these differences do not necessarily impact hip range of motion. This is especially relevant given the recent interest in femoroacetabular impingement as a source of hip and low back pain in young athletes. Femoroacetabular impingement, described as abnormal contact between the femoral head/neck junction and the anterior lip of the acetabulum, is associated with pain and decreased range of motion on hip internal rotation [43–45]. Therefore, it should not be presumed to be "normal" if a young athlete presents with differences in dominant and nondominant hip rotational range of motion as this may be an indicator of hip pathology requiring further attention [41].

Thus careful attention to history and physical exam must be taken in examining the young tennis athlete complaining of hip pain. Hip pain associated with decreased hip internal rotation, pain with internal and external hip rotation, or a history of a "snapping" or "clunking" hip should raise suspicion of intraarticular hip pathology and warrant consideration of advanced imaging with MRI.

Effect of Playing Surface on Hip and Knee Injuries

Tennis is unique in that athletes commonly play on vastly different surfaces with frictional properties that place varying levels of stress on the hip and knee. Research has shown that there is a decreased rate of lower extremity injury on surfaces that allow for sliding (clay) compared to hard court surfaces (asphalt) [46, 47], although the overall rate of early match retirement due to injury in professional tennis was found to be equal between hard court and clay court surfaces [48]. Biomechanical studies have demonstrated surface-based differences in knee flexion during approach to the ball. Hard court surfaces with a higher coefficient of friction were associated with greater knee flexion than clay surfaces where the athlete is able to slide [49]. Thus play on hard court surfaces places greater eccentric stress on the extensor mechanism during knee flexion. This could be one reason for the observed high rates of chronic patellofemoral pain and injuries to the extensor mechanism in tennis athletes.

There have been no known analogous studies to the effects of playing surface on the biomechanics of the hip. However, it would be expected that surfaces with decreased friction would lead to an increased risk for adductor strains while sliding with the legs in abduction.

Risk Factors for Lower Extremity Injuries

In order to adequately address injury prevention in tennis athletes, it is essential to identify risk factors for injury. In a 2-year prospective study of 55 young tennis athletes, Hjelm et al. determined that the only statistically significant risk factor for injury in tennis was existence of a previous injury [50]. Playing greater than 6 h of tennis a week was associated with increased back pain but did not lead to increased rates of injuries to the lower extremities. These findings confirm previous investigations that showed no difference in injury rate based on sex or level of play [7, 9]. The association between sustaining a previous injury and developing a new injury has led some to suggest that injury risk increases with inadequate rehabilitation and treatment of old injuries [50]. By allowing young athletes to return to sport prior to full rehabilitation, they may be at increased risk to reinjury or may make adjustments to compensate for the previous injury that leads to new injury from altered biomechanics.

Conclusion

In conclusion, the young tennis athlete is subject to a unique profile of lower extremity injuries. In the knee, chronic overuse injuries to the patellofemoral compartment and extensor mechanism predominate. The most frequent acute knee injuries are sprains to ligamentous structures, with injuries to the medial meniscus and ACL being most prevalent. In the hip and groin, the most common injuries are adductor strains. Less is known regarding intraarticular injuries to the hip and its surrounding stabilizing structures, although recent research into hip rotation has begun to shed light on intraarticular hip pathology. The biomechanics of hip morphology and range of motion and their relationship to injury in tennis is a growing field that requires further study. There have been recent attempts to identify risk factors for injuries that have demonstrated a link between having sustained an old injury and developing a new injury, although more work is required on this matter. Currently, researchers have a relative grasp of the incidence and types of injuries to the hip and knee that occur in tennis. Future research should be directed toward further elucidation of the risk factors for developing such injuries in order to help tennis athletes avoid future injury.

References

1. Pluim BM, Staal JB, Windler GE, Jayanthi N. Tennis injuries: occurrence, aetiology, and prevention. Br J Sports Med. 2006;40(5):415–23.
2. Reece L, Fricker P, Maguire K. Injuries to elite young tennis players at the Australian Institute of Sports. Aust J Sci Med Sport. 1986;18:11–5.
3. Winge S, Jorgensen U, Lassen Nielsen A. Epidemiology of injuries in Danish championship tennis. Int J Sports Med. 1989;10:368–71.
4. Lanese RR, Strauss RH, Leizman DJ, et al. Injury and disability in matched men's and women's intercollegiate sports. Am J Public Health. 1990;80:1459–62.
5. Hutchinson MR, Laprade RF, Burnett QM, Moss R, Terpstra J. Injury surveillance at the USTA Boys' Tennis Championships: a 6-yr study. Med Sci Sports Exerc. 1995;27(6):826–30.
6. Hahn T, Foldspang A. Prevalent knee pain and sport. Scand J Soc Med. 1998;26(1):44–52.
7. Sallis RE, Jones K, Sunshine S, et al. Comparing sports injuries in men and women. Int J Sports Med. 2001;22:420–3.
8. Silva RT, Takahashi R, Berra B, et al. Medical assistance at the Brazilian juniors tennis circuit–a one-year prospective study. J Sci Med Sport. 2003;6:14–8.
9. Jayanthi N, Sallay P, Hunker P, et al. Skill-level related injuries in recreational competition tennis players. Med Sci Tennis. 2005;10:12–5.
10. Hjelm N, Werner S, Renstrom P. Injury profile in junior tennis players: a prospective two year study. Knee Surg Sports Traumatol Arthrosc. 2010;18(6):845–50.
11. Abrams GD, Renstrom PA, Safran MR. Epidemiology of musculoskeletal injury in the tennis player. Br J Sports Med. 2012;46(7):492–8.
12. Hootman JM, Dick R, Agel J. Epidemiology of collegiate injuries for 15 sports: summary and recommendations for injury prevention initiatives. J Athl Train. 2007;42(2):311–9.
13. Weinstein SL, Flynn JM. Lovell and Winter's pediatric orthopedics. Vol 2, Ch. 28: limb length discrepancy. Lipincott Williams & Wilkins; Philadelphia, PA 2006.
14. Ogden JA, Southwick WO. Osgood-Schlatter's disease and tibial tuberosity development. Clin Orthop Relat Res. 1976;116:180–9.
15. Panattoni GL, D'amelio P, Di stefano M, Isaia GC. Ossification centers of human femur. Calcif Tissue Int. 2000;66(4):255–8.
16. Fabricant PD, Hirsch BP, Holmes I, et al. A radiographic study of the ossification of the posterior wall of the acetabulum: implications for the diagnosis of pediatric and adolescent hip disorders. J Bone Joint Surg Am. 2013;95(3):230–6.
17. Weinstein SL, Flynn JM. Lovell and Winter's pediatric orthopedics. Vol 2, Ch. 23: developmental hip Dysplasia and dislocation. Lipincott Williams & Wilkins; Philadelphia, PA 2006.
18. Kibler WB, Safran MR. Musculoskeletal injuries in the young tennis player. Clin Sports Med. 2000;19(4):781–92.
19. Kibler WB, Safran M. Tennis injuries. Med Sport Sci. 2005;48:120–37.
20. Collado H, Fredericson M. Patellofemoral pain syndrome. Clin Sports Med. 2010;29(3):379–98.

21. Renström AF. Knee pain in tennis players. Clin Sports Med. 1995;14(1):163–75.
22. Fulkerson JP. Patellofemoral pain disorders: evaluation and management. J Am Acad Orthop Surg. 1994;2(2):124–32.
23. Gecha SR, Torg E. Knee injuries in tennis. Clin Sports Med. 1988;7(2):435–52.
24. Rutland M, O'connell D, Brismée JM, Sizer P, Apte G, O'connell J. Evidence-supported rehabilitation of patellar tendinopathy. N Am J Sports Phys Ther. 2010;5(3):166–78.
25. Hak DJ, Sanchez A, Trobisch P. Quadriceps tendon injuries. Orthopedics. 2010;33(1):40–6.
26. Ducher G, Cook J, Spurrier D, et al. Ultrasound imaging of the patellar tendon attachment to the tibia during puberty: a 12-month follow-up in tennis players. Scand J Med Sci Sports. 2010;20(1):e35–40.
27. Kujala UM, Kvist M, Heinonen O. Osgood-Schlatter's disease in adolescent athletes. Retrospective study of incidence and duration. Am J Sports Med. 1985;13(4):236–41.
28. Pihlajamäki HK, Mattila VM, Parviainen M, Kiuru MJ, Visuri TI. Long-term outcome after surgical treatment of unresolved Osgood-Schlatter disease in young men. J Bone Joint Surg Am. 2009;91(10):2350–8.
29. Micheli LJ, Kocher MS. The pediatric and adolescent knee: Ch. 17 tendonopathy of the extensor apparatus of the knee. W B Saunders Company; Philadelphia, PA 2006.
30. Strauss EJ, Kim S, Calcei JG, Park D. Iliotibial band syndrome: evaluation and management. J Am Acad Orthop Surg. 2011;19(12):728–36.
31. Majewski M, Susanne H, Klaus S. Epidemiology of athletic knee injuries: a 10-year study. Knee. 2006;13(3):184–8.
32. Powell JM, Kavanagh TG, Kennedy DK, et al. Intra-articular knee injuries in racquet sports. A review of 128 arthroscopies. Surg Endosc. 1988;2:39–43.
33. Frank JB, Jarit GJ, Bravman JT, Rosen JE. Lower extremity injuries in the skeletally immature athlete. J Am Acad Orthop Surg. 2007;15(6):356–66.
34. Millar AP. Strains of the posterior calf musculature ('tennis leg'). Am J Sports Med. 1979;7:172–4.
35. Delgado GJ, Chung CB, Lektrakul N, et al. Tennis leg: clinical US study of 141 patients and anatomic investigation of four cadavers with MR imaging and US. Radiology. 2002;224:112–9.
36. Kulund DN, Mccue FC, Rockwell DA, Gieck JH. Tennis injuries: prevention and treatment. A review. Am J Sports Med. 1979;7(4):249–53.
37. Perkins RH, Davis D. Musculoskeletal injuries in tennis. Phys Med Rehabil Clin N Am. 2006;17(3):609–31.
38. Akutagawa S, Kojima T. Trunk rotation torques through the hip joints during the one- and two-handed backhand tennis strokes. J Sports Sci. 2005;23(8):781–93.
39. Anderson K, Strickland SM, Warren R. Hip and groin injuries in athletes. Am J Sports Med. 2001;29(4):521–33.
40. Sanchis-Moysi J, Idoate F, Izquierdo M, et al. Iliopsoas and gluteal muscles are asymmetric in tennis players but not in soccer players. PLoS One. 2011;6, e22858.
41. Ellenbecker TS, Ellenbecker GA, Roetert EP, Silva RT, Keuter G, Sperling F. Descriptive profile of hip rotation range of motion in elite tennis players and professional baseball pitchers. Am J Sports Med. 2007;35(8):1371–6.
42. Vad VB, Gebeh A, Dines D, Altchek D, Norris B. Hip and shoulder internal rotation range of motion deficits in professional tennis players. J Sci Med Sport. 2003;6(1):71–5.
43. Safran MR. Evaluation of the hip: history, physical examination, and imaging. Oper Tech Sports Med. 2005;13:2–12.
44. Kelly BT, Weiland DE, Schenker ML, Phillippon MJ. Arthroscopic labral repair in the hip: surgical technique and review of the literature. Arthroscopy. 2005;21:1496–504.
45. Schenker ML, Martin R, Weiland DE, Philippon MJ. Current trends in hip arthroscopy: a review of injury diagnosis, techniques and out- come scoring. Curr Opin Orthop. 2005;16:89–94.

46. Bastholt P. Professional tennis (ATP tour) and number of medical treatments in relation to type of surface. Med Sci Tennis. 2000;11(40):981–990.
47. Nigg BM, Segesser B. The influence of playing surfaces on the load on the locomotor system and on football and tennis injuries. Sports Med. 1988;5(6):375–85.
48. Breznik K, Batagelj V. Retired matches among male professional tennis players. J Sports Sci Med. 2012;11(2):270–8.
49. Damm L, Low D, Richardson A, Clarke J, Carré M, Dixon S. The effects of surface traction characteristics on frictional demand and kinematics in tennis. Sports Biomech. 2013;12(4):389–402.
50. Hjelm N, Werner S, Renstrom P. Injury risk factors in junior tennis players: a prospective 2-year study. Scand J Med Sci Sports. 2012;22(1):40–8.

Chapter 11
Foot and Ankle Injuries in the Young Tennis Athlete

Steven B. Weinfeld

Foot and ankle injuries are quite common in tennis athletes. These include Achilles tendon injuries, ankle sprains and fractures, metatarsal fractures, midfoot sprains (Lisfranc), as well as forefoot injuries including turf toe. Plantar fasciitis and stress fractures also occur commonly in this population. Tennis participation places increased stresses on the foot and ankle due to the acute start and stop nature of the sport as well as sudden changes of direction. Foot and ankle injuries may be prevented by use of proper conditioning techniques, appropriate bracing and shoe wear, and stretching exercises before playing.

Achilles Tendon Injuries

Achilles tendon injuries are very common in tennis athletes. The starting and stopping as well as change of direction required to compete in tennis places the Achilles under tremendous stress. Acute Achilles ruptures are often seen in tennis players. The player feels a sudden pain in the back of the ankle and feels as if they were "struck" in the back of the leg. Players often report hearing a "pop" as well. Immediate pain and inability to ambulate indicate possible Achilles tendon rupture. Examination of the area reveals a palpable defect in the Achilles tendon, most often occurring 4–6 cm proximal to the insertion of the Achilles on the calcaneus. A positive Thompson test (Fig. 11.1) can help confirm the diagnosis. Treatment of acute Achilles rupture usually is surgical repair. Some authors have recently recommended nonsurgical treatment of Achilles rupture [1, 2]. With either method, the tennis athlete is usually sidelined for at least 6–9 months before returning to play. Surgical repair is performed with a modified Krackow locking

S.B. Weinfeld, MD
Foot and Ankle Service, Mount Sinai Medical Center, New York, NY, USA
e-mail: steven.weinfeld@mountsinai.org

© Springer International Publishing Switzerland 2016
A.C. Colvin, J.N. Gladstone (eds.), *The Young Tennis Player: Injury Prevention and Treatment*, Contemporary Pediatric and Adolescent Sports Medicine,
DOI 10.1007/978-3-319-27559-8_11

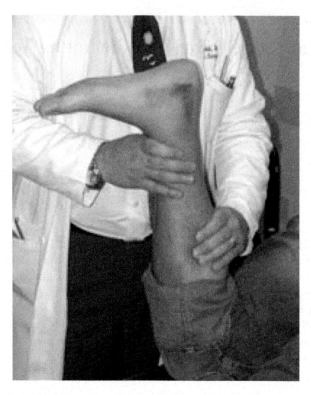

Fig. 11.1 Thompson test indicating a complete rupture of the Achilles tendon. When calf is squeezed and no plantar flexion occurs, the test is positive

suture using #2 nonabsorbable braided suture material. The repair site is then oversewn using a running locking suture with size O absorbable material. Careful repair of the paratenon brings added blood supply to the repair site and minimizes the risk of adhesion of the skin to the underlying tendon. The skin is repaired using nylon sutures. The leg is immobilized in a bulky cotton dressing with plaster strips to reinforce the dressing. This is done to ensure proper wound healing. Non-weight bearing is recommended for 3–4 weeks followed by progressive protected weight bearing. The sutures are removed at 10–14 days and the athlete is placed into a cam walker boot brace. Rehabilitation of an Achilles rupture includes a period of immobilization of up to 6 weeks followed by Achilles-strengthening exercises and physical therapy. Care is taken to avoid passive dorsiflexion stretching of the ankle to prevent accidental compromise of the repair. The athlete may begin active ROM exercises as soon as the sutures are removed. Double heel raises begin at 6 weeks to strengthen the gastroc soleus muscle complex. Straight running is permitted at 3 months and cutting training at 4–5 months. Most tennis players are not able to return to competition for at least 9 months following an Achilles rupture. Return to full strength usually requires 12–18 months.

Achilles tendinitis is significantly more common than frank rupture in the young tennis athlete. Players present with pain and swelling in the posterior aspect of the ankle and difficulty with push-off of the affected limb. Examination reveals swelling and thickening of the Achilles tendon associated with pain with resisted plantar flexion. Treatment includes NSAIDs, ice, immobilization in a boot brace, and limited bending of the ankle. This may require several weeks of nonimpact activity. Physical therapy can accelerate recovery and return to play. Platelet-rich plasma injection into the Achilles tendon has become a popular treatment option, although not supported by adequate studies in the literature [3, 4] Cortisone injections should be avoided as this may precipitate frank rupture of the tendon. Surgery is rarely required for Achilles tendinitis in younger patients.

Ankle Sprains

Ankle sprains are likely the most common injury sustained while playing tennis due to the acute changes of direction required. Most ankle sprains are inversion injuries resulting in damage to the lateral ligamentous structures of the ankle. Players with an ankle sprain will present with swelling and tenderness over the lateral aspect of the ankle. It is important to differentiate a sprain from a fracture, and this can be usually done on exam. Patients with a fracture of the fibula will present with point tenderness on the bone, while a sprain will exhibit tenderness anterior and distal to the fibula at the anterior talofibular ligament. Radiographs of the ankle may be necessary to rule out a fracture. MRI may be necessary to determine the extent of the damage to the lateral ligaments and other associated injuries.

Treatment of an acute ankle sprain consists of rest, ice, compression, elevation, and immobilization. Less severe sprains may be treated with taping or bracing with early return to competition, while more severe sprains may require an extended period of time without playing. Physical therapy can facilitate return to tennis by helping to reduce inflammation and strengthening the peroneal muscles to help prevent recurrent injury. Surgery is not indicated in acute ankle sprains; however, chronic ankle instability may require surgical repair of the lateral ligamentous structures. Bracing is usually employed upon return to tennis to prevent recurrent injury. Most players with a prior ankle sprain will utilize an ankle brace permanently to prevent further injury. Some players will use ankle tape or bracing prophylactically to prevent or minimize injuries. A lace-up ankle support is appropriate for this indication as it provides significant support without limiting motion [5].

Ankle Fractures

Ankle fractures can occur during tennis as the foot is susceptible to severe twisting injuries while cutting and sudden directional changes. Fractures are less common than sprains but require much more significant time away from sport. Players with an ankle fracture will present with point tenderness and swelling directly over the bone and require radiographs to determine the extent of injury.

Non-displaced fractures may be treated with cast or brace immobilization, while displaced or unstable fractures are best treated with open reduction and internal fixation. A player with an ankle fracture will require several months of rehabilitation prior to return to competition. Plates and screws used for ankle fracture fixation do not routinely require removal with the exception of syndesmotic fixation screws. The syndesmotic screws should be removed at approximately 4–6 months following initial surgery and should be removed prior to the player returning to competition [6].

Osteochondral fractures are an uncommon injury to the articular surface of the talus that may be seen in a tennis player with a twisting or impact injury. These are best imaged on MRI and often require surgical intervention. Acute treatment includes immobilization and a period of 4–6 weeks non-weight bearing. Osteochondral lesions that are displaced or continue to be symptomatic are treated with arthroscopic debridement and microfracture to induce growth of reparative cartilage. Following arthroscopic debridement, the player is kept non-weight bearing for 6 weeks followed by progressive protected weight-bearing. Return to competition normally requires 5–6 months [7–9].

Metatarsal Fractures

Metatarsal fractures are quite common in tennis players, and most often occur with a sudden inversion injury of the foot, resulting in a fracture of the fifth metatarsal. This is caused by the pull of the peroneus tertius muscle, resulting in an avulsion fracture of the proximal aspect of the fifth metatarsal. Players will present with acute swelling and tenderness over the base of the fifth metatarsal. Radiographs show a fracture of the proximal aspect of the metatarsal. These fractures are almost universally treated nonsurgically. Immobilization with a CAM walker brace or cast is the most common means of treatment for this fracture. The player may be weight bearing as tolerated in the boot. Surgery is indicated only for significantly displaced fractures or those that have not united successfully [10]. It is important to assess these patients for recurrent ankle instability as this may be the cause of the injury resulting in a metatarsal fracture. Patients with a varus hindfoot alignment are also at higher risk for inversion injuries, resulting in metatarsal fractures (Fig. 11.2).

The Jones fracture occurs in the metaphyseal portion of the fifth metatarsal and is associated with a significant risk of nonunion [11]. These fractures are more likely to be treated surgically to avoid prolonged immobilization and allow faster return to sport. Torg [12] has classified this injury and provided guidelines for treatment of this problem fracture. Nonsurgical treatment consists of 4 weeks non-weight bearing in a cam walker boot or cast. Surgical treatment consists of intramedullary screw fixation without direct exposure of the fracture site. Bone grafting is usually not necessary. Weight bearing is permitted at 4 weeks post op.

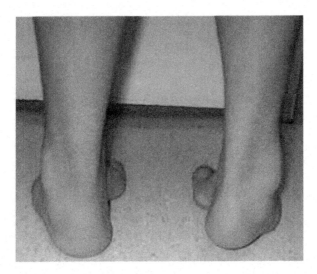

Fig. 11.2 Clinical photo of patient with excessive heel varus predisposing to inversion injuries of the foot and ankle

Fractures of metatarsals other than the fifth metatarsal occur much less frequently and are most often treated with CAM walker or cast immobilization. These are usually stress fractures and will be discussed in that section.

Midfoot Sprains (Lisfranc)

Injuries to the ligaments of the midfoot are also referred to as Lisfranc injuries [13]. This injury occurs at the tarsometatarsal articulation and requires significant force to displace the "Roman arch" of the midfoot (Fig. 11.3). These injuries occur most often with a fixed forefoot while the rest of the limb continues to rotate. A high index of suspicion is necessary to avoid missing these injuries. Patients will present with point tenderness and swelling over the midfoot. Plantar ecchymosis is also an indicator of significant injury to the Lisfranc ligaments. Plain radiographs including oblique views are used to determine displacement and presence of associated fractures (Fig. 11.4). Imaging with a CT scan or MRI is helpful to determine the extent of the injury and to determine appropriate treatment. Truly non-displaced Lisfranc injuries are treated with boot or cast immobilization. Any displacement of the tarsometatarsal joints requires open reduction and internal fixation. This can be done with transarticular screws or plates (Figs. 11.5 and 11.6). Percutaneous pinning should be avoided as the Lisfranc ligaments require at least 12 weeks for healing. Hardware removal should be performed to allow return of motion to the midfoot joints. This should not be done prior to 4 months post surgery to avoid recurrent displacement. Some authors have advocated primary fusion for purely ligamentous injuries to the tarsometatarsal joints [14, 15]

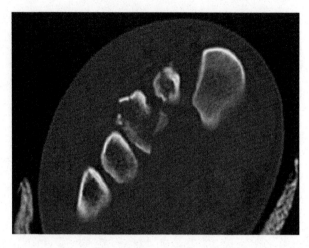

Fig. 11.3 CT scan of patient with Lisfranc fracture and disruption of the "Roman arch" of the midfoot

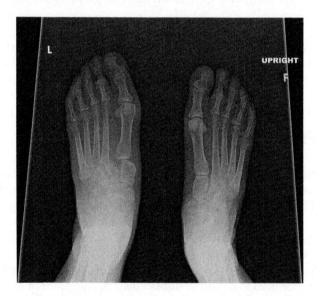

Fig. 11.4 Radiographs of patient with Lisfranc fracture of left foot. Right foot normal midfoot alignment

Forefoot Injuries

The most common forefoot injury in the tennis athlete occurs in the first metatarso-phalangeal joint (MTP). Commonly referred to as turf toe, these injuries include tears of the plantar capsule, ligaments of the first MTP joint, as well as damage to

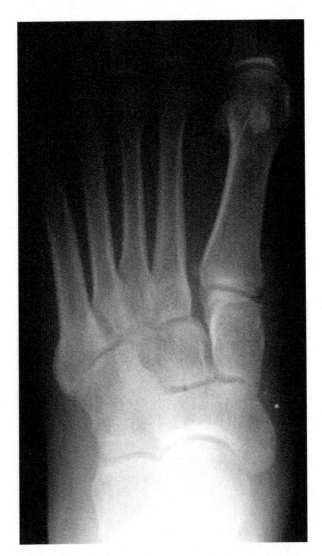

Fig. 11.5 Lisfranc fracture with lateral subluxation of base of second metatarsal base

the sesamoid complex. Hyperextension of the great toe is more often the mechanism of injury causing a traumatic turf toe. Plantar flexion injuries also do occur. Patients with this injury present with swelling and pain in the first MTP joint. Motion of the joint is also painful. Radiographs may be normal and the accurate diagnosis may require imaging with MRI. Treatment consists of a stiff-soled shoe and taping of the toe. A CAM walker boot also is effective at immobilizing the first MTP joint. Surgery is rarely necessary and is indicated for tears of the plantar capsule or sesamoid complex that do not respond to conservative measures.

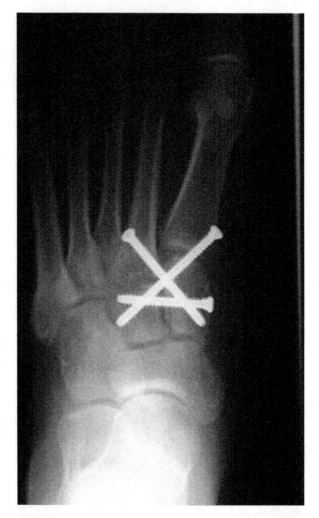

Fig. 11.6 Following ORIF of Lisfranc fracture with screws

Plantar Fasciitis

Plantar fasciitis is a very common disorder seen in tennis players. The plantar fascia is a strong ligament originating from the calcaneus and inserting on the flexor tendons of the toes. It acts as a windlass to help maintain the integrity of the arch of the foot. Inflammation at the origin of the ligament is seen in plantar fasciitis. Patients present with point tenderness on the plantar medial aspect of the heel. Start-up pain when walking as well as morning pain are common complaints. Associated Achilles tightness is common in plantar fasciitis. There is an association with plantar fasciitis and supination of the hindfoot [16]. Acute injury is not usually associated with the development of plantar fasciitis. Diagnosis is made by history and physical examination. Radiographs are most often negative. MRI shows increased signal and thickening of the plantar fascia at its origin. Treatment consists of stretching exercises of the Achilles and plantar fascia, NSAIDs, heel cushions, and orthotics. Cortisone injection may be necessary in patients not improving with the above measures. Care must be taken with using cortisone in this area of the foot as heel fat pad atrophy and frank rupture of the plantar fascia have been described following cortisone injection [17]. Some physicians have advocated the use of platelet-rich plasma (PRP) injection to treat plantar fasciitis; however, further studies are required. Surgical release of the plantar fascia is rarely required and can be performed either open or endoscopically [18]. Surgical treatment should not be considered unless the patient has been treated conservatively for at least 6 months [19].

Stress Fractures

Stress fractures are a frequent problem for the young tennis player. Most commonly, these occur in the metatarsals due to the repetitive stresses of tennis participation. Metatarsal stress fractures usually occur in the diaphyseal part of the bone. Other areas of the foot and ankle where stress fracture may be seen include the calcaneus, distal fibula or tibia, and navicular [20]. Patients will report no history of acute trauma but may have recently increased their playing time or workouts. Swelling and point tenderness are present over the area of stress fracture. Initial radiographs may be normal. Clinical suspicion, along with physical exam, help establish the diagnosis. MRI may be necessary to confirm the presence of a stress fracture. Technetium bone scan also is helpful in establishing the diagnosis. Treatment consists of rest, immobilization, and limited weight bearing. Surgery is rarely indicated [21]. Patients with recurrent stress fractures should be evaluated for a metabolic disorder [22]. Return to tennis is permitted when the fracture site is not tender and healing is evident on radiographs [23]. Foot orthotics may be used to support the foot and ankle to prevent subsequent stress injuries [24]. Can you show an xr and/or mri of stress fx (on xr would not see) and thgen 6 weeks later the callus now seen on XR?

References

1. Soroceanu A, Sidhwa F, Aarabi S, Kaufman A, Glazebrook M. Surgical versus nonsurgical treatment of acute Achilles tendon rupture: a meta-analysis of randomized trials. J Bone Joint Surg Am. 2012;94(23):2136–43.
2. Tan G, Sabb B, Kadakia AR. Non-surgical management of Achilles ruptures. Foot Ankle Clin. 2009;14(4):675–84.
3. Oloff L, Elmi E, Nelson J, Crain J. Retrospective analysis of the effectiveness of platelet-rich plasma in the treatment of achilles tendinopathy: pretreatment and posttreatment correlation of magnetic resonance imaging and clinical assessment. Foot Ankle Spec. 2015.

4. Guelfi M, Pantalone A, Vanni D, Abate M, Guelfi MG, Salini V. Long-term beneficial effects of platelet-rich plasma for non-insertional Achilles tendinopathy. Foot Ankle Surg. 2015;21(3):178–81.
5. Kemler E, van de Port I, Schmikli S, Huisstede B, Hoes A, Backx F. Effects of soft bracing or taping on a lateral ankle sprain: a non-randomised controlled trial evaluating recurrence rates and residual symptoms at one year. J Foot Ankle Res. 2015;8:13.
6. Gardner MJ, Graves ML, Higgins TF, Nork SE. Technical considerations in the treatment of syndesmotic injuries associated with ankle fractures. J Am Acad Orthop Surg. 2015;23(8):510–8.
7. Ahmad J, Jones K. Comparison of osteochondral autografts and allografts for treatment of recurrent or large talar osteochondral lesions. Foot Ankle Int. 2015.
8. Giza E, Delman C, Coetzee JC, Schon LC. Arthroscopic treatment of talus osteochondral lesions with particulated juvenile allograft cartilage. Foot Ankle Int. 2014;35(10):1087–94.
9. Hannon CP, Smyth NA, Murawski CD, Savage-Elliott I, Deyer TW, Calder JD, Kennedy JG. Osteochondral lesions of the talus: aspects of current management. Bone Joint J. 2014;96-B(2):164–71.
10. Smith TO, Clark A, Hing CB. Interventions for treating proximal fifth metatarsal fractures in adults: a meta-analysis of the current evidence-base. Foot Ankle Surg. 2011;17(4):300–7.
11. Hunt KJ, Anderson RB. Treatment of Jones fracture nonunions and refractures in the elite athlete: outcomes of intramedullary screw fixation with bone grafting. Am J Sports Med. 2011;39(9):1948–54.
12. Lehman RC, Torg JS, Pavlov H, DeLee JC. Fractures of the base of the fifth metatarsal distal to the tuberosity: a review. Foot Ankle. 1987;7(4):245–52.
13. Eleftheriou KI, Rosenfeld PF. Lisfranc injury in the athlete: evidence supporting management from sprain to fracture dislocation. Foot Ankle Clin. 2013;18(2):219–36.
14. Sheibani-Rad S, Coetzee JC, Giveans MR, DiGiovanni C. Arthrodesis versus ORIF for Lisfranc fractures. Orthopedics. 2012;35(6):e868–73.
15. Watson TS, Shurnas PS, Denker J. Treatment of Lisfranc joint injury: current concepts. J Am Acad Orthop Surg. 2010;18(12):718–28.
16. Golightly YM, Hannan MT, Dufour AB, Hillstrom HJ, Jordan JM. Foot disorders associated with overpronated and oversupinated foot function: the Johnston County osteoarthritis project. Foot Ankle Int. 2014;35(11):1159–65.
17. Lee HS, Choi YR, Kim SW, Lee JY, Seo JH, Jeong JJ. Risk factors affecting chronic rupture of the plantar fascia. Foot Ankle Int. 2014;35(3):258–63.
18. Nery C, Raduan F, Mansur N, Baunfeld D, Del Buono A, Maffulli N. Endoscopic approach for plantar fasciopathy: a long-term retrospective study. Int Orthop. 2013;37(6):1151–6.
19. DiGiovanni BF, Moore AM, Zlotnicki JP, Pinney SJ. Preferred management of recalcitrant plantar fasciitis among orthopaedic foot and ankle surgeons. Foot Ankle Int. 2012;33(6):507–12.
20. Shindle MK, Endo Y, Warren RF, Lane JM, Helfet DL, Schwartz EN, Ellis SJ. Stress fractures about the tibia, foot, and ankle. J Am Acad Orthop Surg. 2012;20(3):167–76.
21. Weinfeld SB, Haddad SL, Myerson MS. Metatarsal stress fractures. Clin Sports Med. 1997;16(2):319–38.
22. Smith JT, Halim K, Palms DA, Okike K, Bluman EM, Chiodo CP. Prevalence of vitamin D deficiency in patients with foot and ankle injuries. Foot Ankle Int. 2014;35(1):8–13.
23. Meardon SA, Edwards B, Ward E, Derrick TR. Effects of custom and semi-custom foot orthotics on second metatarsal bone strain during dynamic gait simulation. Foot Ankle Int. 2009;30(10):998–1004.
24. Kaeding CC, Yu JR, Wright R, Amendola A, Spindler KP. Management and return to play of stress fractures. Clin J Sport Med. 2005;15(6):442–7.

Erratum to: The Young Tennis Player: Injury Prevention and Treatment

Alexis C. Colvin and James N. Gladstone

Erratum to:

A.C. Colvin, J.N. Gladstone (eds.), The Young Tennis Player: Injury Prevention and Treatment, Contemporary Pediatric and Adolescent Sports Medicine, DOI 10.1007/978-3-319-27559-8

In the content of the 'The Micheli Center for Sports Injury Prevention' pages, the biographies for Dr. Dennis Caine and Dr. Purcell have been removed because they are no longer co-editors for the 'Contemporary Pediatric and Adolescent Sports Medicine' series.

The order of authors in Chapter 10 has been changed to "Steven M. Andelman and Alexis C. Colvin". This has also been updated in the table of contents.

The online version of the original book can be found under
DOI 10.1007/ 978-3-319-27559-8

© Springer International Publishing Switzerland 2016
A.C. Colvin, J.N. Gladstone (eds.), *The Young Tennis Player: Injury Prevention and Treatment*, Contemporary Pediatric and Adolescent Sports Medicine,
DOI 10.1007/978-3-319-27559-8_12

Index

© Springer International Publishing Switzerland 2016   213
A.C. Colvin, J.N. Gladstone (eds.), *The Young Tennis Player: Injury Prevention
and Treatment*, Contemporary Pediatric and Adolescent Sports Medicine,
DOI 10.1007/978-3-319-27559-8

CPSIA information can be obtained
at www.ICGtesting.com
Printed in the USA
BVOW07*1457280816

460368BV00012B/4/P

9 783319 275574